Perioperative Learner's Resource Manual

NANCYMARIE FORTUNATO
RN, BSN, MED, RNFA, CNOR

Perioperative Nursing, Cleveland Clinic Foundation
Cleveland, Ohio

Perioperative Education, Lakeland College
Mentor, Ohio

educator, Educational Services for Professionals
Ashtabula, Ohio

Captain, United States Army Nurse Corps, Reserve Component
Perioperative Nursing OR/HUS
256th Combat Support Hospital
Parma, Ohio

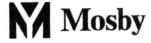

St. Louis Baltimore Boston Carlsbad Chicago Naples New York Philadelphia Portland
London Madrid Mexico City Singapore Sydney Tokyo Toronto Wiesbaden

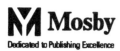

Mosby
Dedicated to Publishing Excellence

A Times Mirror
Company

Publisher: Nancy L. Coon
Acquisition Editor: Michael S. Ledbetter
Senior Developmental Editor: Teri Merchant
Project Manager: Linda McKinley
Manufacturing Supervisor: Linda Ierardi

A NOTE TO THE READER
The author and publisher have made every attempt to check dosages and nursing content for accuracy. Because the science of pharmacology is continually advancing, our knowledge base continues to expand. Therefore we recommend that the reader always check product information for changes in dosage or administration before administering any medication. This is particularly important with new or rarely used drugs.

Copyright © 1996 by Mosby-Year Book, Inc.

All rights reserved. No part of this publication may be reproduced, stored in a retrieval system, or transmitted in any form or by any means, electronic, mechanical, photocopying, recording, or otherwise, without prior written permission from the publisher.

Permission to photocopy or reproduce solely for internal or personal use is permitted for libraries or other users registered with the Copyright Clearance Center, provided that the base fee of $4.00 per chapter plus $.10 per page is paid directly to the Copyright Clearance Center, 27 Congress Street, Salem, MA 01970. This consent does not extend to other kinds of copying, such as copying for general distribution, for advertising or promotional purposes, for creating new collected works, or for resale.

Printed in the United States of America

Printing/binding by Banta Company-Media Center

Mosby-Year Book, Inc.
11830 Westline Industrial Drive
St. Louis, Missouri 63146

International Standard Book Number 0-8151-0827-3
27886

96 97 98 99 00/9 8 7 6 5 4 3 2 1

CONTRIBUTORS

Ruth Bakst, RN, CNOR
Perioperative Educator, St. Luke's Medical Center
Cleveland, Ohio
Educator, Educational Services for Professionals
Ashtabula, Ohio
Registered Nurse Midwife
Capetown, South Africa

Patricia A. Chapek, RN, BA, CNOR
Perioperative Nursing; Cardiac Department, Cleveland Clinic Foundation
Cleveland, Ohio
Educator, Educational Services for Professionals
Ashtabula, Ohio

Nancymarie Fortunato, RN, BSN, MEd, RNFA, CNOR
Perioperative Nursing; Cleveland Clinic Foundation
Cleveland, Ohio
Perioperative Education; Lakeland College
Mentor, Ohio
Educator, Educational Services for Professionals
Ashtabula, Ohio
Captain, United States Army Nurse Corps; Reserve Component
Perioperative Nursing OR/HUS
256th Combat Support Hospital
Parma, Ohio

Katrina E. Hegedus, RN, BSN, CNOR
Perioperative Nurse Manager, MetroHealth Medical Center
Cleveland, Ohio
Educator, Educational Services for Professionals
Ashtabula, Ohio

Susan M. McCullough, RN, BSN, CNOR
Perioperative Nursing, Eye Institute, Cleveland Clinic Foundation
Cleveland, Ohio
Educator, Educational Services for Professionals
Ashtabula, Ohio

Martin A. Phillips III, RN, BSN, CNOR
Director of Perioperative Services, Marymount Hospital
Garfield Heights, Ohio
Captain, United States Army Nurse Corps; Reserve Component
Head Nurse-OR/HUS
256th Combat Support Hospital
Parma, Ohio

PREFACE

The *Perioperative Learner's Resource Manual* is designed to align with the chapter arrangement in *Berry and Kohn's Operating Room Technique, 8th edition*. The purpose of the resource manual is to enhance the use of the main text and offer additional educational information and exercises for the learner. Included in the resource manual are suggested learning objectives, study questions, and critical thinking activities. Each chapter features expanded concepts and new material not included in the main text. Learning objectives and study questions for the new content are also included.

STRUCTURE OF THE PERIOPERATIVE LEARNER'S MANUAL

The *Perioperative Learner's Resource Manual* is intended for use in the classroom and clinical sites. Each chapter opens with an introduction followed by learning objectives derived from the content of the main text and new material included in the resource manual. Competency-based knowledge and skills are identified by learning style. An emphasis on global understanding of "why" and "how" instead of performing tasks without knowing the rationale is stressed throughout.

In Chapter 1 of the main text, the various sources available for learning, gathering information, and continuing education are discussed. Chapter 1 of the resource manual expands on this theme by discussing computer-enhanced literature searches and walks the learner through a simulated search. In addition to personal learning, the variations in learning styles of adults and children are explored. Chapter 2 of the main text focuses on the foundation of patient-centered care in the OR. New material added in Chapter 2 of the resource manual includes a basic discussion of how a nursing environmental theorist established the groundwork for patient care standards in the OR. The emphasis is on the setting of standards and why they are important to the care of the patient. In turn, each chapter of the resource manual is designed to expand on the theme established by the corresponding chapter of the main text. New definitions not included in the main text are added as they apply.

A summary at the end of each chapter ties the content of the main text in with the new material presented in the resource manual. Additional references and resources are listed at the end of each chapter to augment those included in the bibliography of main text.

CONTENTS

SECTION ONE: CORRELATION OF THEORY AND PRACTICE

Chapter 1   Introduction for the Learner, 1
Chapter 2   Foundations of Patient-Centered Care, 6
Chapter 3   Accountability and Professional Obligations, 11
Chapter 4   Legal and Ethical Issues, 15

SECTION TWO: THE PERIOPERATIVE HEALTH CARE TEAM

Chapter 5   The Direct Patient Care Team, 19
Chapter 6   Operating Room Staff and Supporting Services, 21

SECTION THREE: THE PATIENT AS A UNIQUE INDIVIDUAL

Chapter 7   The Patient: The Reason for Your Existence, 23
Chapter 8   Patients with Special Needs, 28

SECTION FOUR: THE SURGICAL ENVIRONMENT

Chapter 9   Physical Facilities, 32
Chapter 10   Potential Sources of Injury to Caregiver and Patient, 35

SECTION FIVE: SURGICAL ASEPSIS, INSTRUMENTATION, AND EQUIPMENT

Chapter 11   Attire, Surgical Scrub, Gowning, and Gloving, 38
Chapter 12   Essentials of Asepsis: Application of Principles of Aseptic and Sterile Techniques, 40
Chapter 13   Sterilization and Disinfection, 42
Chapter 14   Surgical Instrumentation, 44
Chapter 15   Specialized Surgical Equipment, 46

SECTION SIX: PREOPERATIVE PATIENT CARE

Chapter 16   Preoperative Preparation of the Patient, 48

SECTION SEVEN: ANESTHESIA CONCEPTS AND CONSIDERATIONS

Chapter 17   General Anesthesia: Techniques and Agents, 51
Chapter 18   Local and Regional Anesthesia, 53
Chapter 19   Patient Monitoring and Potential Complications Related to Anesthesia, 55

CONTENTS, continued

SECTION EIGHT: INTRAOPERATIVE PATIENT CARE

Chapter 20	Coordinated Roles of Scrub Person and Circulator, 58
Chapter 21	Positioning the Patient, 60
Chapter 22	Skin Preparation and Draping of the Surgical Site, 62
Chapter 23	Hemostasis and Blood Loss Replacement, 64
Chapter 24	Wound Closure Materials, 67

SECTION NINE: POSTOPERATIVE CARE OF THE PATIENT AND ENVIRONMENT

Chapter 25	Surgical Wounds: Factors Influencing Healing and Infection, 69
Chapter 26	Postoperative Patient Care, 75
Chapter 27	Postoperative Care of the Physical Environment, 78

SECTION TEN: SURGICAL SPECIALTIES

Chapter 28	Diagnostic Procedures, 80
Chapter 29	General Surgery, 82
Chapter 30	Gynecologic and Obstetric Surgery, 84
Chapter 31	Urologic Surgery, 86
Chapter 32	Orthopaedic Surgery, 88
Chapter 33	Ophthalmic Surgery, 90
Chapter 34	Plastic and Reconstructive Surgery, 92
Chapter 35	Otorhinolaryngology Surgery: Ear, Nose, and Throat Surgery, 94
Chapter 36	Head and Neck Surgery, 95
Chapter 37	Neurosurgery, 96
Chapter 38	Thoracic Surgery, 97
Chapter 39	Cardiac Surgery, 98
Chapter 40	Peripheral Vascular Surgery, 99

SECTION ELEVEN: MULTIDISCIPLINARY PERIOPERATIVE CONSIDERATIONS

Chapter 41	Ambulatory Surgery, 100
Chapter 42	Perioperative Pediatrics, 102
Chapter 43	Perioperative Geriatrics, 103
Chapter 44	Organ Procurement, Transplantation, and Replantation, 104
Chapter 45	Oncology, 106

SECTION ONE: CORRELATION OF THEORY AND PRACTICE

CHAPTER 1 — INTRODUCTION FOR THE LEARNER

After reading Chapter 1 of the text, the learner should attain the following objectives and competency-based knowledge and skills. Additional learning objectives may be identified by the learner through continued education and literature review. Computer searches are explored in this resource chapter as one method of literature review.

LEARNING OBJECTIVES

- Identify three characteristics of adult learners.
- Name five educational resources available for the learner.
- Contrast effective and ineffective verbal communication.
- Demonstrate nonverbal communication.
- Identify three barriers to learning.

COMPETENCY-BASED KNOWLEDGE

- Understand the difference between andragogy and pedagogy.
- Understand how the nursing process applies to patient teaching.
- Understand how the development of objectives applies to learning as well as patient outcomes.
- Understand why effective communication is essential in the OR.

COMPETENCY-BASED SKILL

- Use available resources for learning.
- Participate in effective communication.
- Apply psychomotor skills to cognitive skills.

UTILIZING COMPUTERS TO UPDATE KNOWLEDGE AND SKILL

Computerization has opened a myriad of opportunities for learners. Current information is as close as an on-line catalog at a library or a telephone line with a modem at home. Many databases have been developed that contain concise information that can be reviewed 24 hours a day through home-based computers. Some databases are accessible for a fee; others are available at no cost. National and international computer services, such as *Prodigy*™, *America Online*™, *CompuServe*™, and *Internet*™, are accessed for a fee based on time of day and duration of hookup.

Many institutions permit employees or designated learners to access an in-house library computer from their own homes utilizing a modem/communication package system at no cost. Most medical institutions have *Medline*™ on CD-ROM. Some may permit access to this database through a home-based modem. Local city and county libraries, including most colleges and universities, permit modem access to on-line catalogs at no charge.

A modem is a communication device that may be contained within the computer as a circuit board or attached to the computer by an electronic cable as a peripheral device. Newer computers, particularly 486 models or higher, including *Pentium*™, have a modem built-in. Modems are available in different speeds called baud rates. The most efficient baud rates (speeds) exceed 9600. It is advisable that the purchaser of a computer with a built-in modem inquire as to the speed of the internal modem system. Often, internal modems are slower than 9600 baud and need to be upgraded. Software (computer communication program) is usually included with the modem that enables it to work. If a built-in modem is present, the software is usually preloaded and the system needs only to be plugged into a phone line to be useable. Most learners affiliated with colleges and universities, as well as their educators, may purchase additional academically priced computer software and hardware at a significant savings over the cost to the general public. Often the savings exceed several hundred dollars.

LEARNING TO PERFORM A LITERATURE SEARCH USING A COMPUTER

Most computer database services have predesigned methods of constructing a computer search. Often a menu system is used that allows the searcher to respond to prompts by questions that appear on the computer screen. The premise for a computer search is based on key words or specific topics. If the terms used in the search are too broad, the information offered by the computer in response will be far more than the searcher can assimilate. Using specific terms helps the computer to be selective in rendering information. Standardized computerized subject headings have been developed and are in use by most major medical databases. The most popular is the *Medical Education Subject Headings* (MESH), which is used by the National Library of Medicine (NLM) in Bethesda, Maryland. An understanding of medical terminology is essential.

The actual questions asked by the computer at the prompts may vary, but the *content* is the same. The computer will be able to narrow down information to a usable level by limiting parameters to years of publication and language desired. Some search programs require the searcher to type in words or select words from built-in lists, such as the MESH. Some search programs incorporate a combination of built-in lists and/or typed-in responses. Most of the search programs are very easy to use and are designed to make searching the literature fun and easy. Specialized systems can allow the searcher to actually read or print selected articles, but most systems are limited to retrieving only the citation. Frequently, abstracts are available and can be printed with the citation. See generic sample search for demonstration of how a computer can offer ways to make a search specific to information desired.

SAMPLE COMPUTER-GENERATED LITERATURE SEARCH

After hookup by a computer modem to a remote computer at a library:

> Information desired by the searcher: *surgical removal of gall bladder.* The MESH term is cholecystectomy. The computer will ask for the subject (from the MESH):
>
> __ **SUBJECT TO BE SEARCHED**_____
>
> The searcher will respond by typing in the appropriate word (from the MESH):
>
> __ **CHOLECYSTECTOMY**
>
> The computer will ask about limits of search:
>
> __ **DO YOU DESIRE TO LIMIT SEARCH TO SPECIFIC YEARS?**
>
> The searcher will respond by typing in the publication years desired:
>
> __ **1991-1996**
>
> The computer will ask if further limits are desired:
>
> __ **DO YOU DESIRE TO LIMIT SEARCH TO A SPECIFIC LANGUAGE?**
>
> The searcher will respond indicating the desired language parameters of the articles or texts. (Some computer search programs will start offering lists to choose from at this point.):
>
> __ **ENGLISH**
>
> The computer will ask if further limits are desired and will specify additional parameters available in the system, such as specific authors or publications (not all parameters are available in all systems):
>
> __ **SHOULD OTHER LIMITS BE APPLIED TO SEARCH?**
>
> *At this point, the searcher will respond to the prompts offered by the computer to indicate additional limits available in the system.*
>
> The computer will ask if the search is ready to be started (or executed):
>
> __ **READY TO START THE SEARCH?**
>
> The searcher will respond by indicating yes or no in the manner requested by the computer:
>
> __ **YES**
>
> The computer will perform the search and place them into a set. The computer will inform the

STUDY QUESTIONS

1. List several methods that can be used to research a subject in the literature. (Refer to Chapter 1 of text.)
2. Write a paragraph comparing andragogy and pedagogy. (Refer to Chapter 1 of resource manual.)

3. Outline the main steps used to perform a literature search using a computer. (Refer to Chapter 1 of resource manual.)
4. Write a paragraph discussing the effects of stress on job performance.

CRITICAL THINKING ACTIVITIES

1. Develop a role-playing scenario demonstrating positive verbal communication (negative verbal communication)
2. Develop a role playing scenario demonstrating positive nonverbal communication (negative nonverbal communication)
3. Compare/contrast the impact of negative communications between caregivers in the presence of patients and their families.
4. Lead a class discussion group based on stress reduction for the caregiver.
5. Prepare a short educational discussion for a group of adults (andragogic approach).
6. Prepare a short educational program for children (pedagogic approach).
7. Construct a sample computer search inquiry based on the sample on page 3. Go to the local library and request assistance from library personnel in performing a computer search.

DEFINITIONS

andragogy Philosophy of teaching adults that allows for individualized flexibility, choice, and modification specific to developmental stage. Utilizes the principles of adult learning.

appendix Section of a text containing useful, additional information to a text, such as charts, tables, graphs, or sample documents. Usually found at the back of a book.

bibliography References used to create a body of text. Can be found after a body of text or at the back of a book.

Bloom's taxonomy Measurement of learning outcomes. This taxonomy is a set of descriptive verbs that classify cognitive and affective domains in a stair step progression starting with basic learning and progressing to complex knowledge in a hierarchical manner.

competency testing Creating scenarios that demonstrate possession of required knowledge and skill to perform a task or solve a problem.

critical thinking Acquiring knowledge, categorizing facts, applying information, making decisions, implementing action, and evaluating outcomes in a real or simulated environment.

glossary Collection of terms to define the authors meaning. They may be found at beginning or end of a chapter or at the back of a book.

index Alphabetized lists of keywords, subjects, and topics found in the back of a book.

inquiry Investigation that seeks truth, knowledge, and facts.

mentor Wise, trusted counselor with whom a learner aligns in a knowledge-sharing relationship.

pedagogy Philosophy of teaching children in an authoritative and preoutlined manner that is specific to developmental stage.

preceptor Instructor who imparts knowledge in an outlined manner. Not always a personalized relationship.

premise A supposition that supports a conclusion.

rationale Fundamental reason for action, belief, or premise.

role model Person who is knowingly or unknowingly imitated by admirer(s). No personalized relationship exists.

SUMMARY OF CHAPTER 1

Adult learners are unique because they need to have control over their acquisition of knowledge. They prefer to have choices and relate concurrent learning to past experiences. The philosophical teaching approach most effective with adults is andragogic. The main difference between adult and child learners is the degree of structure applied to the teaching process. Children require more structure and are less self-directed than adults. The philosophical teaching approach most effective with children is pedagogic.

Acquiring knowledge from other persons, such as mentors, preceptors, or role models, is an acceptable form of learning. Additional knowledge may be gained by accessing material contained in libraries and other sources, such as computer databases. Most systems are easy to use and formal training is not always necessary. Often, easy-to-follow, step-by-step instructions are provided right on the computer screen.

ADDITIONAL RESOURCES

America Online
8619 Westwood Center Drive
Vienna, VA 22182-2285
1-800-827-6364

Delphi International Services Corporation
Internet connection information
1-800-695-4005

National Library of Medicine
On-line literature searching services
1-301-496-4000

National Student Nurse's Association
555 West 57th Street
New York, NY 10019
1-212-581-2211

Prodigy Services Company
22 North Plains Industrial Highway
Wallingford, CT 06492
1-800-776-3449

CHAPTER 2 — FOUNDATIONS FOR PATIENT-CENTERED CARE

The origin of perioperative patient care standards is explored in this chapter. The premise for the roles of the perioperative nurse and the surgical technologist is identified by the practice standards established by their professional organizations, Association of Operating Room Nurses (AORN) and Association of Surgical Technologists (AST). Understanding and participating in standard-setting groups empower caregivers in control of professional practice issues. Chapter 3 of this resource manual discusses involvement with standard-setting groups through an exploration of group dynamics.

Perioperative nurses apply the nursing process in the development of the plan of care. The standards for this process are established by the American Nurses' Association (ANA). As a licensed, registered professional, the perioperative nurse is accountable for the coordination and implementation of the plan of care for the patient in the perioperative environment. This includes a certain amount of accountability for the delegation of patient care activities to other caregivers. In the OR, the perioperative nurse and the surgical technologist work together in concert with other OR team members for the benefit of the patient. Although the roles of caregivers may differ, the desire for positive patient outcomes is a common theme.

LEARNING OBJECTIVES

- Identify the phases of the perioperative experience.
- List the components of the nursing process.
- Identify three sources of patient care standards.

COMPETENCY-BASED KNOWLEDGE

- Discuss the assessment phase of the nursing process.
- Discuss development of the nursing diagnosis.
- Discuss the planning phase of the nursing process.
- Discuss the importance of outcome identification.
- Discuss the implementation phase of the nursing process.
- Discuss the evaluation phase of the nursing process.

COMPETENCY-BASED SKILL

- Outline the relationship between the patient and the perioperative nurse.
- Outline the relationship between the patient and the surgical technologist.
- Outline the relationship between the patient and the environment.
- Outline the relationship between the caregiver and the environment.
- List three methods of documenting patient care.

ORIGIN OF PATIENT CARE STANDARDS

Nursing theorist, Florence Nightingale (1820-1910), is credited with developing the environmental theory of patient care. (See Box 2-1, Nightingale's Theory of Nursing.) According to the theory, the caregiver provides the best environmental conditions possible to prevent unnecessary suffering and to allow nature's reparative processes to take their course.

BOX 2-1

NIGHTINGALE'S THEORY OF NURSING		
PHYSICAL ENVIRONMENT	**PSYCHOLOGIC ENVIRONMENT**	**SOCIAL ENVIRONMENT**
Sanitation Ventilation Lighting Noise Odors Temperature	Communication Advice Variety Scientific knowledge base Creativity Spirituality	Mortality data Prevention of disease Education of caregiver Nursing is distinct from medicine Accountability Responsibility

This involves manipulating the environment through proper sanitation, ventilation, and hygiene. Nightingale's theory is the cornerstone for the standards of perioperative patient care still in effect today (See Box 2-2, Standards of Care Established by Florence Nightingale.) Manipulation of the environment serves as protection for both the patient and the caregiver. She emphasized the need for prevention through education and teamwork. In her eyes, the team consisted of not only the caregivers, but also the patient and his or her family. She prepared the family, as well as the caregiver, for the patient's ongoing needs. In her theory, everything and everyone are part of the environmental influence.

BOX 2-2

STANDARDS OF CARE ESTABLISHED BY FLORENCE NIGHTINGALE
Sanitation: Protects the patient and the caregiver from infection
Lighting: Sets the mood, illuminates the surgical site to facilitate a safe procedure.
Warmth: Normothermia is critical to homeostasis and comfort of the patient and the caregiver.
Ventilation: Proper air handling in the OR benefits the patient and the caregiver.
Effluvia: Characteristic odors have psychologic influence; some odors signal hazardous conditions.
Noise: Characteristic sounds have a psychologic impact on the patient and the caregiver; some sounds may be distracting, others may be soothing.

Nightingale, as a naturalist, viewed the environment as an external force that influenced the well-being of the patient by preventing, suppressing, or contributing to disease or death. Naturalistic and holistic care is merged in the plan of care, viewing the whole patient and his or her family from every aspect. Standards of her day are still observed in operating rooms throughout the world. The Nightingale pledge outlines standards for personal and professional attributes of the caregiver (See Box 2-3, Nightingale Pledge). She also stressed that nursing was an art and a science. She frequently approached her legislators with suggestions for bills and laws designed to protect patients and caregivers.

Nightingale felt that minimal competency should be attained before entering into practice. Her training programs were the first competency-based nursing education offered to caregivers. She stressed that an increased level of practice required an increased level of education. Credentialling, such as licensure or certification, should be time-limited and subject to renewal periodically. Although her program taught only the basics, she supported her student's efforts in pursuing continuing education and specialty training.

BOX 2-3

THE NIGHTINGALE PLEDGE

I solemnly pledge myself before God, and in the presence of this assembly, to pass my life in purity and to practice my profession faithfully.

I will abstain from whatever is deleterious and mischievous, and will not take or knowingly administer any harmful drug.

I will do all in my power to maintain and elevate the standard of my profession, and will hold in confidence all personal matters committed to my keeping and all family matters coming to my knowledge in the practice of my profession.

With loyalty, will I endeavor to aid the physician in his work, and devote myself to the welfare of those committed to my care.

Developed by Lydia E. Gretter, RN, and the planning committee for the 1893 graduating class of the Farrand Training School, now known as Harper Hospital, Detroit, Michigan.

STUDY QUESTIONS

1. What are the phases of the perioperative experience?
2. What are the components of the nursing process?
3. What does scope of practice mean?
4. What is the difference in the educational preparation of the perioperative nurse and the surgical technologist?
5. What is competency?
6. What is credentialling?
7. What is a standard?

CRITICAL THINKING ACTIVITIES

1. Write a simulated plan of care for a patient having an exploratory laparotomy.
2. Write a simulated plan of care wherein the evaluation is modified because of an unknown condition discovered at the time of the surgical procedure.
3. Simulate a role playing scenario wherein the caregiver interviews the patient.
4. Participate in a community awareness program based on educating the public about the roles of operating room personnel.

SUMMARY OF CHAPTER 2

Professional registered perioperative nurses and surgical technologists work together as a team for the benefit of the patient. Although the plan of care is developed by the registered nurse, the surgical technologist is integral in the implementation and on-going evaluation of the outcomes.

Standards are developed by professional organizations as practice manuallines. Medical, nursing, and technical organizations design standards specific to the type of practice parameters encompassed by the scope of permitted practice. Patterning practice attributes after the standards helps to ensure that the caregiver is attempting to render safe, responsible, and efficient patient care.

Credentialling is a form of regulation extended by governmental or private agencies. Governmental agencies provide licensure under appropriate circumstances for physicians and nurses. Licensure is a measure of minimal competency. Private organizations provide certification and validate knowledge and skill through testing. Certification is a measure of knowledge and achievement above minimal competency.

The origin of patient care standards has its foundation in the environmental theories of Florence Nightingale. She was the first to believe in the art and science of nursing and to work for validating the practice of patient care through her writings, teachings, and later, her legislative proposals.

ADDITIONAL RESOURCES

Agency for Health Care Policy and Research (AHCPR)
P.O. Box 8547
Silver Spring, MD 20907
1-800-358-9295

American National Standards Institute (ANSI)
11 West 42nd Street
New York, NY 10036
1-212-642-4900

Association for the Advancement of
Medical Instrumentation (AAMI)
3330 Washington Boulevard, Suite 400
Arlington, VA 22201-4598
1-703-525-4890

American Nurses Association (ANA) Publications
P.O. Box 90660
Washington, DC 20090-0660
1-800-637-0323

American Hospital Association (AHA)
1 North Franklin
Chicago, IL 60606
1-312-422-3000

Association of Operating Room Nurses (AORN)
2170 South Parker Road, Suite 300
Denver, CO 80231-5711
1-800-755-4676

Association of Surgical Technologists (AST)
7108-C South Alton Way
Englewood, CO 80112-2106
1-800-637-7433

Joint Commission on Accreditation of
Healthcare Organizations (JCAHO)
One Renaissance Boulevard
Oakbrook, IL 60181
1-708-916-5600

National Certification Board:
Perioperative Nursing (NCB:PNI)
2170 South Parker Road, Suite 295
Denver, CO 80231-5711
1-303-369-9566

Sigma Theta Tau International
550 West Worth Street
Indianapolis, IN 46202
1-317-634-8171

ADDITIONAL READING

Nightingale F: *Notes on nursing: What it is, and what it is not,* New York, 1969, Dover Publications.

Gruendeman BJ, Fernsebner B: *Comprehensive perioperative nursing: Volume One: Principles,* Boston, 1995, Jones and Bartlett Publishers.

Roth RA: *Perioperative nursing core curriculum,* Philadelphia, 1995, W.B. Saunders Co.

CHAPTER 3   ACCOUNTABILITY AND PROFESSIONAL OBLIGATIONS

Professionalism is reflected in the relationships and activities between the patient, the physician, and the caregiver. Patients seek medical care from reliable sources and trust that the personnel rendering care are professional and competent. Patient satisfaction is a measurable outcome directly related to competency in terms of proficiency and efficiency. Caregivers should value the trust placed in them by the patient. This trust and confidence are the main premises for the plan of care.

Collaboration between the patient and caregivers in the development of the plan of care is an important aspect of advocacy. This concept is strengthened by the desire of the caregiver to uphold and support the patient's rights and wishes in the delivery of care. The patient has the right to determine the extent of care given under all circumstances. It is both a duty and a responsibility to honor the wishes of the patient, despite personal biases. Caregivers need to examine their own belief systems and have an understanding of how personal feelings affect patient care. Additionally, caregivers need to understand how the environment and interpersonal/interprofessional relationships affect performance.

Standards, policies, procedures, and other manuallines for patient care are established by professional organizations, workplace committees, or governmental regulatory/accreditation bodies. Although the intent of professional manuallines is grounded in the desire for safe, efficient patient care, care providers are expected to perform within the parameters with minimal margin of variation. Chapter 2 of this resource manual discussed the conceptual origin of patient care standards. This resource chapter explores involvement with group process as a way to participate in setting standards of practice.

LEARNING OBJECTIVES

- List five patient rights from the American Hospital Association's (AHA) "Patient's Bill of Rights".
- List three main aspects of accountability.
- List three main aspects of patient advocacy.
- Identify the main components of informed consent.
- Identify the purpose of advance directives.
- Discuss the implications of consent for a surgical procedure.
- Discuss how the work environment affects performance.
- Discuss the importance of standardization.
- Describe how group process influences the setting of standards.

COMPETENCY-BASED KNOWLEDGE

- Understand the relationship between professionalism and accountability.
- Understand the impact of patient advocacy on patient care.

- Understand how personal feelings could possibly influence care delivery.
- Understand the importance of collaboration with the patient in the plan of care.
- Understand how group process influences the establishment of standards.
- Understand how standardization facilitates proficient and competent care.

COMPETENCY-BASED SKILL

- Apply standards to care delivery.
- Serve as a patient advocate.
- Demonstrate the ability to locate and utilize available practice manuals and manuals.

THE IMPORTANCE OF GROUP PROCESS IN SETTING STANDARDS

Standards of care are established by groups of professionals in the interest of maintaining high levels of performance and results in a particular area of practice. Standards are derived through a collaborative effort brought about through the group process. The members of the group share examples, research, and experiences. The care delivery process is compared with the desired outcome, and a standard is identified.

Types of standards that are developed by professional groups include:
- Process standards to outline the procedures for patient care and caregiver activities.
- Content standards to outline specific criteria.
- Outcome standards to outline the desired result of care.
- Interdisciplinary standards to outline interaction between various types of patient care providers.

Understanding the workings of the group process may encourage future involvement with standard-setting groups and/or regulatory agencies. Involvement with professional organizations allows the caregiver to lend a voice to professional practice parameters. This can provide performance enrichment, job satisfaction, and patient satisfaction.

From earliest recorded history, standard setting and decision making took place in groups. This was important because the standards had to be applied and adhered to by the entire population in order to be effective. Essentially, core groups set the pace for the rest of the population. In modern times, establishing standards on a national or institutional level still requires the work and brainpower of a core group (AKA: committee). The development of feasible standards depends on the cohesive, creative, and productive qualities of the group. By nature, humans are group-seeking beings, which accounts for the type of group structures seen at all levels of personal and professional activities. Becoming active at the group or committee level enables the caregiver to have a voice in setting the ground rules for practice. An understanding of how groups work can make involvement with a standard-setting committee more productive, participative, and professionally satisfying. Having a voice in the foundation of practice empowers the professional with the ability to control the workplace environment and the work product itself.

In order to have a productive standard-setting committee, a series of events need to take place. These events are collectively referred to as *group dynamics*. Group dynamics involve coordinated actions comprising of interpersonal communication, a sense of belonging, interdependency, mutual goals, equality, and motivation. Because each personality differs to varying degrees, a series of structured roles and relationships emerges. Usually, groups that are called together for a specific purpose have a designated leader. However, other members of the group may assume this role for temporary periods of time. On the other hand, a group that forms naturally, without specifically being called together, develops a spontaneity unique unto itself. One or more persons share the responsibility for the leadership functions in an alternating pattern or in partnership. Naturally forming groups may become functional and productive faster because the group dynamics originate with cohesiveness and a common bond. It is interesting to note that groups that are called together take varying lengths of time to produce results. According to Bruce Tuckman (1965), groups need to take the time for *forming* and getting to know and trust each other. Functional activity patterns need to be established, referred to as *norming*, before they begin to process information. Norms cannot be imposed, but develop out of the needs and personalities of the group members. There may be some degree of power shifting known as *storming* before the group can start *performing* in unison. The final act of the group is *adjourning*. Closure, as natural process, takes place after the completion of the mission of the group is attained.

The working mission of the group should be clearly established during the forming and norming stages and reinforced frequently during the storming phase by the leader(s). Keeping a clear perspective of the mission will help override personal interests and political scenarios that hinder productivity. With the mission in the forefront, the group is better able to perform at peak efficiency. The experience of working through the progressive stages of group process is professionally satisfying, giving the participants a sense of accomplishment.

STUDY QUESTIONS

1. How does peer pressure affect performance?
2. What are the main points regarding the patient's consent for a surgical procedure?
3. Does the patient have the right to get off the OR table and refuse treatment? Discuss this situation in essay form.
4. How are data from performance improvement studies used to change the delivery of patient care?
5. How does a committee work together to set standards?

CRITICAL THINKING ACTIVITIES

Volunteer to serve on an established committee within the institution. Caregivers can join intra- or interdepartmental groups organized for specific purposes, such as policy & procedure, standards, peer evaluation, or other topic. Some groups are permanent, such as performance improvement, others are temporary, such as an employee party planning group. Learners can serve on school committees. The purpose for serving on a committee is to learn how to have a voice in creating and maintaining the work environment. Patient care issues are frequently identified and the standard of care is determined. Involvement in the group process, beginning at a social level (employee party planning group) and working toward a complex decision-making group (policy setting group), enables the caregiver or learner to participate in setting the pace for the work or learning environment.

DEFINITIONS

accountability The responsibility of a person or group to answer to another person or group for actions taken or not taken.

advance directives The documentation of written decisions of a patient regarding his or her care in the event of inability to make treatment decisions for self. This is a legal document that incorporates durable power of attorney and living wills.

  durable power of attorney The legal designation of a person who is authorized by the patient to make decisions on his or her behalf in the event he or she becomes incapacitated.

  living will The written legal wishes of the patient in regards to the refusal of treatment or extent measures to prolong life.

advocacy The support given to the patient and family by the caregiver.

competency The level of performance is appropriate and in accordance with acceptable standards of care.

informed consent The recipient of care is apprised and acknowledges understanding of a sequence of events as it may benefit or potentially cause injury in the course of permitted therapy or treatment.

obligation The sense of duty to or a binding promise to perform appropriately and in the best interest of the patient and the team.

standardization The uniformity in performance of procedures.

SUMMARY OF CHAPTER 3

Accountability is the duty to respond appropriately to a series of obligations to both the patient and other caregivers. Accountability and professional performance are derived from standard levels of activity, whether it is in the provision of patient care or interaction with coworkers. Everyone in the workplace has rights. Some rights are established by professional agencies; others are incorporated into state or federal laws.

Standards are at the heart of professional practice. Understanding what standards are and becoming involved with standard-setting groups provides an opportunity to exercise control over patient care issues.

ADDITIONAL READING

Bandman EL: *Critical thinking in nursing, ed 2;* Norwalk, CT; 1995, Appleton & Lange.

Jacono BJ, Jacono JJ: In my opinion: A holistic approach to teaching responsibility and accountability, *Nurse Educator* 20(1):20-23, 1995.

Long L: *Understanding/Responding: A communication manual for nurse, ed 2;* Boston; 1992, Jones and Bartlett.

Mason EJ: *How to write meaningful standards of care,* Albany, NY, 1994, Delmar Publishers, Inc.

Poulton BC: Setting standards of care, *Nursing Standard* 8(51):3-13, 1994.

Snowdon AW, Rajacich D: The challenge of accountability in nursing, *Nursing Forum* 28(1):5-11, 1993.

CHAPTER 4   LEGAL AND ETHICAL ISSUES

Competent patient care is the best way to avoid the dilemma of a malpractice claim. Unfortunately, even under the best of circumstances a patient may suffer an injury and recover monetary damages as compensation. Understanding how a malpractice claim starts and how it proceeds is important in the effort to avoid the many pitfalls that can lead to being named in a lawsuit.

LEARNING OBJECTIVES

- List the 4 Ds of malpractice.
- Define negligence as it relates to caregivers.
- Discuss the level of responsibility a caregiver has for his or her own actions.
- List three important features of OR documentation.
- Discuss the process of going through a deposition.

COMPETENCY-BASED KNOWLEDGE

- Understand how negligence can lead to tort action.
- Understand the difference between following orders of a superior and responsibility to patient.
- Understand the importance of appropriate documentation of patient care.
- Understand the difference between a standard and a recommended practice.
- Understand how performance is measured against standards in legal situations.
- Understand how conscience and personal bias could influence care delivery in a bioethical situation.

COMPETENCY-BASED SKILL

- Demonstrate competency in documentation of patient care and outcomes.
- Identify three potential events that could lead to a lawsuit.
- Explain three doctrines upon which lawsuits may be based.
- Discuss two universal moral principles that guide ethical decision making.

DEPOSITION

Any caregiver, despite due caution in practice, may be named in a lawsuit. Physicians and those with "larger pockets" are generally named in lawsuits more often than nonphysician caregivers (nurses and technicians). However, nonphysician caregivers may be named if the plaintiff is advised that the employer (institution or private practice) can be held liable for the employee's actions. Being named in a lawsuit is not necessarily an accusation of wrong doing. When a patient sustains an injury, all persons who came in contact with the patient, regardless of job status, will be named in the suit. The burden of proof is placed on the plaintiff to show that someone's negligent act caused the injury. Usually, primary defendants are identified, but other people brought in are examined as witnesses and considered potentially liable. This process is called the discovery phase. In the case of *Res Ipsa Loquitor (the thing speaks for itself)*, the burden of proof rests with the defense to show they were not negligent and did not cause the injury.

Part of the discovery process includes a sworn statement under oath, which is referred to as a *deposition*. All parties involved with a lawsuit will undergo a deposition, or be "deposed". This helps both sides of the argument determine if the case should be brought to a courtroom setting. Each deponent will have the opportunity to review the charted documentation and relevant facts of the case before being deposed. Each deponent will be questioned by both the plaintiff's attorney and the defendant's attorney. All statements are recorded by a court recorder and printed in a bound transcript for presentation to each attorney. The deponent will have the opportunity review the contents of the transcript and sign that the statements are accurate as recorded before the case goes to trial. In some cases, after the discovery process is complete, a monetary settlement for damages may be reached before the case ever goes to trial.

During the deposition, the attorneys will have the opportunity to object to specific questions for the record, but the deponent will still be required to respond. This objection is recorded to flag questions that are to be ruled on by the judge at a later date and/or to alert the deponent to potentially tricky questions. Questions may be phrased in compound sentences intended to cause the deponent to answer with long explanations. This is desirable to the plaintiff's attorney because the content of the deposition may be read to the jury during the trial. Damaging conclusions could be drawn from misspoken or emotion-driven testimony. If the deponent feels a surge of emotion, he or she has the right to request a break in the proceedings rather than to answer in haste. Simple "yes" or "no" answers are the least inflammatory answers. Be cautious of overgeneralized questions. They could be used to illustrate a parallel scenario that is not truly part of the event in question and may create a credibility issue.

The main points to remember if called to give a deposition are:
- A summons to appear will be issued.
- Each deponent the right to personal legal counsel in addition to one supplied by the employer.
- Follow the advice of legal counsel regarding conversations about the potential case.
- An updated curriculum vitae (résumé) may be requested for the record during the deposition.
- Review the documentation the patient's care.
- Review policies, procedures, state regulations, and professional standards of practice.
- Tell the truth in response to questions by the attorneys.
- Avoid giving opinions. Discuss only the facts as requested.
- Don't volunteer information not solicited.
- "I don't know" or "I don't remember" are acceptable responses if the deponent is uncertain of the facts in question.
- Short answers are in order; preferably "yes" or "no".
- If a narrative answer is required, be brief. Ask the questioning attorney to break down compound questions so the responses may be specific and to the point.
- Any records or personal notes are subject to examination by the attorneys if their existence is discovered during the deposition.

After all parties involved with a potential lawsuit have been deposed, the case may be presented at trial. The parties, who were deposed, will be called to the stand at the trial and questioned, much in the same way they were questioned during the deposition. The questions may relate to the information brought out in the deposition or new material that surfaces during questioning of other witnesses. During the trial, if one of the attorneys raises an objection to a question, the judge rules on whether the witness is to respond or not. The trial proceedings are recorded for permanent record by a court reporter. The transcripts are then a matter of public record.

Avoiding a successful lawsuit involves documentation of competent performance within the standard of care. This means being knowledgeable about policies and procedures. It also means maintaining skill through continued education. Becoming active in professional organizations is one way to remain current with new developments and trends in patient care.

The most common causes for malpractice lawsuits naming nonphysicians are:
- Falls
- Foreign body left in patient
- Medication errors
- Injury by faulty or misused equipment
- Failure to monitor the patient's condition
- Not informing physician of change in patient's condition
- Invasion of privacy/breach of confidentiality

STUDY QUESTIONS

Match column A to column B. Each term is used only once.

A		B
1	Tort	_____ Optimal behavioral objectives
2	Liability	_____ Leaving a patient who needs care
3	Negligence	_____ Professional misconduct, lack of judgment or skill
4	Abandonment	_____ What a prudent caregiver would do in a similar circumstance
5	Incident report	
6	Standard	_____ A wrong that causes injury to another person
7	Ethics	_____ Adverse outcome
8	Malpractice	_____ Situation involving morals, values, or beliefs
9	Injury	_____ Report of irregular occurrence
10	Recommended practice	_____ Legally responsible for damages
		_____ Lack of care or skills

CRITICAL THINKING ACTIVITIES

1. Attend a meeting of the institution's bioethics committee. Create a case study based on a bioethical situation and how the role of the bioethics committee could interface with decision making.

2. Conduct a class discussion about the relationship between *Res Ipsa Loquitor* and the burden of proof. Upon whom does the burden of proof fall in this circumstance? Explain why.

DEFINITIONS

causation An action directly or indirectly caused an injury.
damages Monetary compensation awarded to make restitution for an injury, wrong, or a harm.
    compensatory damages Awarded recompense for a proven injury.
    punitive damages Awarded in excess of compensatory damages as a form of punishment.
defendant The person(s) named in a lawsuit.
deposition Sworn statement given under oath.
    deponent Person who gives sworn statement under oath for the record.
plaintiff The person(s) who initiates a lawsuit. Must prove that the defendant failed to perform in the same way a reasonable and prudent person of the same status would perform in the same or similar circumstances.
statute of limitations An affixed time period wherein a plaintiff may bring a lawsuit against a potential defendant. The time period varies according to state law. Special extended time periods may exist wherein minors may have to a specified age (differs by state), considered the age of reason, to initiate a lawsuit.

SUMMARY OF CHAPTER 4

All caregivers are subject to potential lawsuits. The key thing to remember is that each person is responsible for his or her own actions. Innocent people may be named in a suit without consequence. These people are usually called as witnesses and may be questioned by both defense and plaintiff attorneys in an effort to discover the facts surrounding the event. Being named in a suit is not always an accusation of negligence or malpractice.

ADDITIONAL READINGS

Association of Operating Room Nurses: *Ethical dilemmas in perioperative nursing,* Denver, CO, 1990.

Feutz-Harter S: *Nursing and the law*, ed 4, Eau Claire, WI, 1991, Professional Education Systems, Inc.

Fiesta J: *20 legal pitfalls for nurses to avoid*, Albany, NY, 1994, Delmar Publishers, Inc.

Gifis SH: *Law dictionary*, Hauppauge, NY, 3rd ed, 1991, Barron's Educational Series.

SECTION TWO: THE PERIOPERATIVE HEALTH CARE TEAM

CHAPTER 5 — THE DIRECT PATIENT CARE TEAM

Each intraoperative caregiver contributes to the plan of care in role-specific ways. Each role is important to the attainment of expected outcomes. Chapter five of the main text discusses each intraoperative role briefly, along with educational requirements and licensure issues. Nurses and physicians are state licensed and regulated. Surgical technologists and physicians assistants are not. State legislature is vague for unlicensed personnel, but does create a role delineation to prevent unlicensed personnel from practicing the role of a licensed caregiver. Performing in the role of a physician or nurse carries a state-regulated penalty.

Unlicensed personnel practice according to standards created by their professional organizations and other governing bodies, such as the American Medical Association (AMA), and guidelines set by national organizations, such as the Joint Commission on Accreditation of Healthcare Organizations. Unlicensed assistive personnel may provide some direct patient care under the supervision of a registered nurse. The nurse is responsible for delegating only those tasks for which the assistive person is capable of perform in a safe and competent manner. Competency is grounded in knowledge and skill gained from training and clinical practice.

LEARNING OBJECTIVES

- Identify members of the operating room team.
- Know the difference between sterile and unsterile team members.
- Compare the differences between the scrub and circulator role.
- Identify personnel who perform in the role of first assistant.
- Identify personnel responsible for the administration of anesthesia.

COMPETENCY-BASED KNOWLEDGE

- Define the concept of sterile team.
- Define the concept of unsterile team.

COMPETENCY-BASED SKILL

- Perform in the role of a sterile team member according to performance description.
- Perform in the role of a nonsterile team member according to performance description.

COMPETENCY IN PERFORMANCE

Competence is the documented ability to understand the rationale behind a specific function and perform that function in accordance with established and accepted practice standards.

Identification of expected competencies assists the registered nurse in the utilization and evaluation of unlicensed assistive personnel. The expected competencies may vary between practice settings, but should be closely aligned with the state's nurse practice act and regulations set forth by other governing bodies. Periodic performance testing is recommended to assure supervisory personnel of competent performance in all employees.

In 1985, the Association of Operating Room Nurses (AORN) adopted a competency model consisting of 18 competency statements that identify knowledge, skill, and ability as being hallmarks of competent perioperative nursing practice. Each statement provides a means by which to measure performance and achievement in each competency can be documented. The National Certification Board: Perioperative Nursing, Inc. (NCB:PNI) has also established the importance of knowledge and skill in the description of competent practice. More recently, in 1994, AORN approved *Perioperative Advanced Practice Nurse Competency Statements* based on curriculum guidelines created by the National Organization of Nurse Practitioner Faculties.

The validation of competent practice is important to all caregivers. Assistive personnel, professional nurses, and advanced practice nurses alike are expected to provide knowledgeable, skillful, and appropriate care according to established standards of practice for their role.

STUDY QUESTIONS

	Place a S in front of the sterile team members and a U in front of the unsterile team members
Sterile team member	___ circulator
	___ scrub person
	___ first assistant
Unsterile team member	___ second assistant
	___ surgeon
	___ anesthesia provider

CRITICAL THINKING ACTIVITIES

1. Construct a list of key elements of working together as a team. Consider the differences in each team member's role and how each person can make a contribution to the plan of care.
2. Diagram the physical position of each team member during the intraoperative phase of care. Use separate colors to indicate sterile areas from nonsterile areas.

DEFINITIONS

anesthesia provider An anesthesiologist or a certified registered nurse anesthetist

SUMMARY OF CHAPTER 5

Each caregiver's role is vital to the patient's attainment of expected outcomes. Competency in that role is monitored by measurable criteria set forth by professional organizations and regulating bodies. Competency is based on knowledge, skill, and ability.

CHAPTER 6   OPERATING ROOM STAFF AND SUPPORTING SERVICES

LEARNING OBJECTIVES

- Identify the roles of indirect caregivers in and out of the OR.
- Discuss how committees are important for the coordination of activities in the OR.

COMPETENCY-BASED KNOWLEDGE

- Understand the importance of a job description (performance description).
- Delineate the role distinction between the managerial and educational coordinators in the OR.
- Delineate the role distinction between an advanced nurse practitioner and staff registered nurse in the OR.
- Compare the roles of surgical technologist and licensed practical/vocational nurse in the OR.

COMPETENCY-BASED SKILL

- Identify Three preoperative patient care areas.
- Identify Two postoperative patient care areas.
- Identify Three perioperative areas involved with patient testing.
- Identify Three supporting services used in perioperative patient care.
- Demonstrate communication with indirect patient care supporting service departments.
- Discuss how committees influence the delivery of patient care.

INTRAOPERATIVE COORDINATION OF SPECIALTY SUPPORT SERVICES

Cooperation between indirect patient care disciplines is the hallmark of well-coordinated support services. It is especially important that these services be performed in a timely fashion for efficient patient care during the surgical procedure. Although all support services are important for patient care, the x-ray and biomedical departments have a unique role and are often in demand on a 24-hour basis.

An x-ray technician should have equipment set up and in position before the patient enters the OR. The x-ray technician's role includes performing scout films to identify landmarks or locate foreign bodies and intraoperative radiographs as required. This technician is also responsible for fluoroscopy equipment (C-arm), its settings, and operation. The technicians enforce safety by instructing the surgical team to use protective shields and lead aprons appropriately and announce when the equipment is activated and emitting x-rays.

Biomedical technicians maintain OR equipment and ensure its functionality and safe operation. They may perform last-minute electrical safety checks of new equipment preoperatively or make repairs of complex items such as lasers, electrosurgical units, or physiologic monitoring equipment. More extensive repairs are usually performed in a workshop away from the OR. Replacement equipment brought in on loan at night when in-house equipment fails is thoroughly checked by biomedical personnel before being placed into service.

The 24-hour availability of x-ray personnel and biomedical technicians is important for efficient patient care during regular business hours and off-hours emergencies. Larger teaching facilities may have these personnel in-house at all times. Smaller facilities frequently have one or two specialty technicians in-house during business hours, but use an "on call" system to accommodate emergency procedures after hours. At night, the OR team performing emergency surgery assesses the need for supporting services and activates the after hours call in protocol.

STUDY QUESTIONS

Identify which caregiver is responsible for each patient care activity. Refer also to Chapter 5 of the main text. Place the letter of the role in front of the patient care activity or performance description.

1. Nurse practitioner
2. Perfusionist
3. Registered nurse
4. Nursing assistant
5. X-ray technician
6. Biomedical technician
7. Environmental services
8. Clinical educator
9. Materials manager
10. Scrub person

____ Develops and activates the plan of care
____ Passes sterile instruments to surgeon
____ Performs intraoperative radiographs
____ Orders supplies
____ Conducts inservice programs
____ Performs advanced nursing procedures
____ Nonnurse personnel who help with patient care
____ Maintains and repairs OR equipment
____ Runs cardiopulmonary bypass machinery
____ Cleans the OR

DEFINITIONS

job description (performance description) A written summary of role and criteria by which to measure performance of that role.

SUMMARY OF CHAPTER 6

Support services and indirect patient care personnel have important roles in the global performance of perioperative patient care.

ADDITIONAL RESOURCES FOR SECTION TWO

National Organization of Nurse Practitioner Faculties, *Advanced nursing practice: Nurse practitioner curriculum guidelines,* Washington, DC, 1990.

SECTION THREE: THE PATIENT AS A UNIQUE INDIVIDUAL

CHAPTER 7   THE PATIENT: THE REASON FOR YOUR EXISTENCE

Each patient has a unique set of characteristics that define personality, physical attributes, and interaction with the environment. Some of these unique characteristics are based on age, sex, ethnicity, and health status considerations. Caregivers who develop the perioperative plan of care for a particular patient often have limited time for interviewing. Having a standardized baseline from which to start can be helpful in eliminating the need to rediscover some of the things that are common to most humans during particular stages of life. These are known as developmental stages. If during the assessment the caregiver finds that the patient is not at an expected developmental stage, then the assessment pattern changes. Modifications to standardized assessment are individualized for each patient. These are the components upon which the perioperative caregiver can focus for a more "instant rapport".

Health assessment and treatment can be placed on a more finite level by the use of algorithms. An *algorithm* is a step-by-step, flowchart-like method of examining a set of data, especially data regarding a health status consideration. Algorithms also incorporate alternative solutions or pathways that can be used to problem solve, predict responses, and/or interpret data. The end result is the outcome, much like that incorporated in the plan of care in the form of expected outcomes. Figure 7-1 shows a sample algorithm for perioperative patient care.

The combination of developmental stage assessment and the use of algorithms enables the caregiver to assess the patient as an individual according to unique and standardized formats.

LEARNING OBJECTIVES

- Identify characteristics of a patient-centered approach in perioperative care.
- Identify the patient's basic needs according to Maslow's Hierarchy.
- Discuss how adaptive processes are used by patients during the perioperative experience.
- Discuss how intrinsic stress factors influence the patient's expected outcomes.
- Discuss how extrinsic stress factors influence the patient's expected outcomes.

COMPETENCY-BASED KNOWLEDGE

- Understand the need for individualization in patient care.
- Understand how adaptation affects attainment of expected outcomes.
- Understand how the patient perceives care.

COMPETENCY-BASED SKILL

- Create an individualized plan of care for a perioperative patient.

- Perform interventions to reduce the patient's anxiety and fear in the perioperative environment.
- Communicate effectively with the patient's family and significant others.

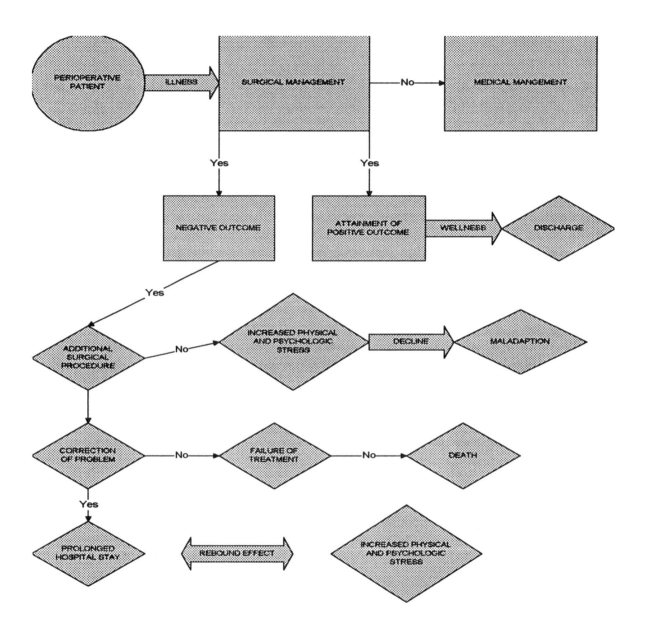

FIGURE 7-1
SAMPLE PERIOPERATIVE PATIENT EXPECTED OUTCOME
ALGORITHM

USING DEVELOPMENTAL THEORY TO UNDERSTAND THE PATIENT'S UNIQUENESS

Developmental theorists have studied human growth, motivational issues, and behavioral responses through many disciplines. Psychoanalytic theorists observe personality traits and attribute exhibited behavior to mental or psychic condition. These behaviors are motivational, defensive, and controlling influences that affect how a person perceives and responds to a situation. Behavioral theorists, who also practice a form of psychotherapy, describe actions according to cognitive (understanding) and affective (response) processes. Cognitive theorists, on the other hand, maintain that a person's thoughts determine how he or she perceives and responds. These theories are closely intertwined, but care is taken not to categorize patients by how we think they perceive a situation. Objective observation reveals their responses but not subjective feelings. The discipline from which a developmental theory is derived may vary, but once the theory is applied to an individual patient, that patient continues to remain unique, despite similarities to other patients.

Patients who present to the OR for a surgical procedure may have more than one medical diagnosis. They also have a set of personal beliefs and behaviors that may modify an expected response to the perioperative experience. In combination, these factors make the patient one of a kind. Certain parameters, validated by scientific studies, can be used to estimate potential responses. Developmental theorists base their theories on biologic, chronologic, motivational, and stair-step stages that have been demonstrated in large proportions of the population. These are more or less considered norms, but should not be thought of as absolutes. Table 7-1 shows examples of developmental theories and the progressive or regressive direction a patient's behavior may take.

STUDY QUESTIONS

Match term from column A with definition in column B

A		B
1. Expected outcome	_____	Inner belief in higher power
2. Plan of care	_____	Physiologic and psychologic change as a defense mechanism
3. Hierarchy of needs	_____	Low level of self care
4. Adaptation	_____	Emotion marked by dread
5. Anxiety	_____	Reject reality
6. Dependency	_____	Individualized physiologic and psychologic response to situation
7. Denial	_____	Maslow's concept of patient priorities
8. Coping	_____	Identified result of an action
9. Fear	_____	Apprehensive uneasiness
10. Spiritual need	_____	Outline of interventions based on assessment

CRITICAL THINKING ACTIVITIES

Create a sample plan of perioperative care based on a developmental theory. Use the computer search method discussed in Chapter 1 of this resource manual. Suggested key words include: *the name of the theorist, the name of the theory,* human development, stage theory, and hierarchy. Other search terms may lead to additional data from which to construct a developmental plan. Consider limiting the search to manageable parameters, such as sex or age.

DEFINITIONS

algorithm A systematic method of evaluating a patient's condition to effect appropriate treatment.

SUMMARY OF CHAPTER 7

Although, the patient's baseline assessment is compared with an expected set of norms, data gathered may deviate according to individual developmental issues. Personality, morals, motivation, values, and in some ways, cognition change in concert with life-stages. Some patients will be in tune with the norms for their chronologic age and others will lag behind or surpass expectations. The unique differences necessitate individualization of the plan of care so the patient may attain a positive outcome.

Table 7-1 Examples of Developmental Theories

Theorist	Parameter	Features of theory	Patient response	Other considerations
Erikson	Biologic/Chronologic stair-step progression of personality stability	Continuum closely related to age based on behaviorism, psychoanalysis, and humanistic theories.	Unfinished developmental issues can be taken to the next stage.	Measures positive and negative responses of both sexes through the life span.
Havighurst	Developmental tasks / vectors	Certain life processes should be accomplished by certain ages.	Some patients have interruptions in the processes and experience maladaption as a result.	Ranges from infancy to later maturity for both sexes.
Jung	No formal stages, but progression is chronologic. Based only on adults, not children.	Balances introversion with extroversion. Humanistic.	Inner yearning for a sense of a higher power.	Based on 10-15 adult archetypes, rather than childhood behaviors. Differs between males and females.
Kohlberg	Measures level of moral reasoning by age levels	Move through three levels of moral development progressing in six stages from internalized ideas to externalized actions.	Progresses through "Me," "Others," and "Us" stages of relationships based on internal versus external rewards.	Can stop progressing at any time. May remain in a low, selfish level or progress to higher, selfless level. Based on a male model.
Kubler-Ross	Stages of grief. Usually found at close of life regardless of age. Based on cognitive and affective status.	Progressive steps to positive state of normative grief. Adaptive process.	Progress through denial, anger, bargaining, depression, up to acceptance.	Can experience two stages at once. Time elements vary. Pathologic grief occurs if person is stuck in a stage and cannot move forward. Family and significant other experiences the stages at their own pace, also.
Loevinger	Stairstep hierarchy of personality/ego development by stages, not age-related	Move through 10 step hierarchy as the result of a conflict or value judgment.	Lower levels of hierarchy are self gratuitous. Higher levels are more sophisticated and moral.	May get stuck in a conformist state and have difficulty moving forward.
Maslow	Motivational theory based on humanistic theories of need	Needs are defined as deficiency (D needs) or being (B needs). D needs are basic to life and survival (physical & safety issues). B needs are basic to psychologic well-being (love, esteem, & self-actualization). B needs are met after D needs have been filled.	Unsatisfied D needs can lead to negative outcomes. Unsatisfied B needs can lead to psychologic void.	These are identified throughout the life span. Self-actualization is the highest attainment. May be reached at various stages of life in a temporary or permanent state. Motivation to attain B or D needs causes the movement through the levels.
Piaget	Cognitive theory	Cognition is based on sensorimotor, preoperational, concrete, and formal aspects of becoming a thinking adult.	Process of thought process development from birth to late teen years.	Final stage attained as older teenager is carried through adulthood.

CHAPTER 8 PATIENTS WITH SPECIAL NEEDS

Assessment of the patient with multiple health status considerations involves a more complex analysis. The baseline assessment should start by establishing the patient's developmental stage, but take into consideration that physical health may cause a maladaptive effect. Physical illness has a major impact on how the patient progresses or regresses through the stages of development. The patient may manifest a combination of deviations from the expected norms. Behaviors can range from hostility to depression. Some may seem passive and disinterested. Patients who are assessed in a perioperative setting usually have one or more medical diagnoses (comorbidity) that interface with their developmental stages and evoke responses to the current situation. This can be confusing if the patient is expressing his or her feelings in an unexpected or unacceptable manner. When assessing a patient in the perioperative setting, consider that he or she is in an unaccustomed environment under the influence of physical and psychologic stressors. Patients with compound medical diagnoses, also referred to as special needs patients, frequently experience maladaptive responses to the surgical experience. Caregivers need to understand this phenomenon and modify their assessment strategies to accommodate the patient's individuality.

LEARNING OBJECTIVES

- Identify specific patient populations that have special needs.
- Identify health status considerations that may alter the patient's response to the surgical experience.

COMPETENCY-BASED KNOWLEDGE

- Understand how health status considerations can affect the assessment of the patient's developmental stage.
- Understand how patients cope with complex medical diagnoses.

COMPETENCY-BASED SKILL

- Demonstrate skill in the individualized preoperative assessment of a patient with multiple medical diagnoses.
- List several deviations in coping mechanisms that may be employed by perioperative patients with complex medical diagnoses.

COPING MECHANISMS OF SPECIAL NEEDS PATIENTS

Psychologic defenses help all patients cope with fearful or stressful situations. Coping mechanisms develop to meet a specific need. Types of coping mechanisms used vary according to developmental stage and the level of perceived threat. Different mechanisms are more acceptable at certain ages. For example, behavior enacted by a small child is less acceptable when habitually displayed by an adolescent. Temporary behaviors that would seem inappropriate for the patient's expected developmental stage are sometimes part of an adaptive process. As the patient adapts to a change in health status so does the need to rely on coping mechanisms. Eventually, the patient adapts and uses fewer defenses. Patients who have difficulty adapting to declining health also have difficulty coping. They may use various coping skills inappropriately in a pathologic sense. Table 8-1 lists several common coping mechanisms.

TABLE 8-1 Common Coping Mechanisms

Mechanism	Meaning	Objective Assessment	Example
Denial	Rejects responsibility. Unable or unwilling to accept the truth	Stammers, may or may not make eye contact, seems to be making excuses	"I do not have lung cancer"
Displacement	Shifting blame to a weaker substitute	Submissive to power figures, but critical and oppressive to subordinates	"My doctor never tells me anything. The lab must be wrong"
Identification	Acts like an admired hero or villain	Outward signs of indecisiveness and low self-esteem	"My sister and I both feel ill. We both have the same disease, I'll bet"
Projection	Attributing unacceptable behavior to others	Acts suspicious of others, defensive posture	"The cigarette manufacturer enticed me to smoke"
Rationalization	Justifying behavior with plausible statements	May be defensive or smug. Trying to save face. Can become hostile	"I only became ill because cancer runs in my family"
Reaction formation	Acts differently than he or she feels inside	Confusion, irrational. Mood swing. May seem overly conscientious and moral	"These are not tears of sadness. They are tears of joy because I will be dead soon"
Regression	Revert to a more primitive state of being	May assume closed, fetal position. Crossed arms and legs, looking downward, crying. Prolonged silences	"I want my mother"
Repression	Blocks unacceptable thoughts and feelings	Blank stare, questioning look. No in-depth discussions	"I don't remember what my diagnosis is. Why am I here?"

STUDY QUESTIONS
Circle True or false
1. True or false   Developmental stages all depend on chronologic age.
2. True or false   Hearing impaired patients must remove hearing appliances before coming to the OR.
3. True or false   Verbal communication, in elevated tones, is more direct for mentally impaired patients.
4. True or false   Patients with nutritional deficiencies are at risk for impaired skin integrity.

5. True or false   Metabolic disturbances do not influence wound healing.
6. True or false   Stress can increase blood glucose levels.
7. True or false   Neurovascular disease predisposes a patient to pressure injury.
8. True or false   Obese patients may be malnourished.
9. True or false   Obese patients often have two or more medical diagnoses.
10. True or false   Visually impaired patients benefit from wearing visual aids to the OR.
11. True or false   Pregnancy is a contraindication for local anesthesia.
12. True or false   Preterm labor is a possible complication of surgical intervention.
13. True or false   The enlarging pregnant uterus can alter anatomic landmarks by displacement of abdominal organs.
14. True or false   In maternal hemorrhage, blood naturally shunts toward the pregnant uterus.
15. True or false   Fetal viability is measured by body weight and lung maturity.
16. True or false   Maternal laboratory values are consistent with the average nonpregnant adult.
17. True or false   Immunosuppression increases the patient's risk for wound infection.
18. True or false   An HIV-positive mother can pass the virus to her unborn fetus.
19. True or false   A single positive HIV test is confirmation of the disease AIDS.
20. True or false   Terminally ill patients cope at their own developmental levels.

CRITICAL THINKING ACTIVITIES

Create a sample plan of care for a perioperative patient with multiple diagnoses, such as pregnancy, obesity, and diabetes. Incorporate as many diagnoses as possible. Find the common thread between the physical and psychologic components. Alter the patient's profile by changing age or sex. Combine this plan with the critical thinking exercise in Chapter 7.

DEFINITIONS

comorbidity A combination of illnesses or maladaptive states, which may include two or more mental or physical disorders simultaneously

coping mechanisms Psychologic defenses used by an individual to reduce levels of anxiety, fear, shame, or painful feelings. This is an unconscious, automatic reaction to a perceived threat.

SUMMARY OF CHAPTER 8

Patients with comorbid conditions are at increased risk for complications in the perioperative environment. Appropriate assessment and the subsequent development of a plan of care specific to the patient's needs can prevent or minimize many problems that can be attributed to having a surgical procedure. Assessment includes the physical and psychologic aspects that make each patient unique. The perioperative nurse, who identifies the nursing diagnoses and expected outcomes, should incorporate allowances for developmental stage and coping skills. Caregivers should consider the whole patient and his or her interaction with the environment when planning and implementing interventions. The evaluation of the plan is demonstrated by the positive attainment of desired and expected outcomes.

ADDITIONAL RESOURCES FOR SECTION THREE

National Institutes of Health
9000 Rockville Pike
Clinical Center, Bldg. 10, #2C206
Bethesda, MD 20892
(301) 496-0441

National Institute of Mental Health: Public Inquiries Section
5600 Fishers Lane
Rockville, MD 20857

Society for Health and Human Values
6728 Old McLean Village Drive
McLean, VA 22101
(703) 556-9222

ADDITIONAL REFERENCES

Bohlander JR: Differentiation of self: An examination of the concept, *Issues in Mental Health Nursing* 16(2):165-184, Mar-Apr 1995.

Corey G: *Theory and practice of counseling and psychotherapy*, ed 4, Belmont, CA, 1991; Brooks/Cole Co.

Critchley DL: *Psychiatric and mental health nursing with children and adolescents*, Gaithersburg, MD; 1992, Aspen.

Dixon J et al: Psychometric and descriptive perspectives of illness impact over the life span, *Nursing Research* 40(1):51-56, Jan-Feb 1991.

Freiberg KL: *Human development: A life-span approach*, ed 4, Boston; 1992, Jones & Bartlett.

Haber J et al: *Comprehensive psychiatric nursing*, ed 4, St Louis, 1992, Mosby-Year Book.

Hayes RL: The legacy of Lawrence Kohlberg: Implications for counseling and human development, *J of Couns & Devel* 72(3):261-267, Jan-Feb 1994.

Kelleher K: The afternoon of life: Jung's view of the tasks of the second half of life, *Perspec Psych Care* 28(2):25-28, Apr-Jun 1992.

MacLean TB: Influence of psychosocial development and life events on the health practices of adults, *Issues in Mental Health Nurs* 13(4):403-414, Oct-Dec 1992.

Nkongho NO: Teaching health professionals transcultural concepts, *Holistic Nursing Practice* 6(3):29-33, Apr 1992.

Pender NJ: Expressing health through lifestyle patterns, *Nursing Science Quarterly* 3(3):115-122, Fall 1990.

Ulrich YC: Gender differences: Implications for understanding woman's development, *Kansas Nurse* 68(4):1-2, Apr 1993.

Vessy JA, Richardson BL: A holistic approach to symptom assessment and intervention, *Holistic Nursing Practice* 7(2):13-21, Jan 1993.

SECTION FOUR: THE SURGICAL ENVIRONMENT

CHAPTER 9 — PHYSICAL FACILITIES

Surgical procedures were not always performed under optimal conditions in controlled environments. Understanding the modern surgical suite and its adjunct areas is important for the maintenance of traffic flow and infection control. Learners may want to organize personal knowledge and skill objectives according to Table 9-1.

TABLE 9-1 Environmental Considerations

Knowledge	Skill
Zones within suite	Identifying potential problems
Microbiology, transmission	Aseptic technique
Universal precautions	Infection control
Environmental Parameters	Wearing appropriate attire
Standards and recommended practices	Surgical conscience
Policy and procedure	
Regulating agencies	

LEARNING OBJECTIVES

- Identify specific areas within the OR suite wherein attire and behaviors affect the manner of care delivery.
- Discuss how the practice of surgery moved from private homes to institutional settings.

COMPETENCY-BASED KNOWLEDGE

- Understand how environmental layout contributes to aseptic technique.
- Understand how individual caregivers can support an aseptic environment.
- Understand how atmospheric controls contribute to an aseptic environment.

COMPETENCY-BASED SKILL

- Demonstrate appropriate traffic flow patterns incorporating common areas, limited access areas, and peripheral support areas.

HISTORICAL BACKGROUND OF HOSPITAL-BASED PATIENT

Medical care has its roots in superstition and magic. Primitive humans believed that supernatural and/or evil forces caused illness and death. Conversely, they believed that the same forces could be used to reverse adverse effects. Most of the spiritual manipulation was performed by a central leadership figure, such as a medicine man or healer. In some societies this was done in a ritualistic fashion or as part of a religious rite by chanting prayers or casting spells. Surgical care, on the other hand, was more barbaric in origin and was first performed without benefit of anesthesia, with the rare exception of alcoholic beverages. The emphasis was placed on physical strength and speed, rather than precision. Most surgical procedures were performed by unskilled, untrained persons. The ancient Indians and Greeks were ahead of their time in technique and instrumentation, but not until the seventeenth and eighteenth centuries did major advances leading to more scientific techniques take place.

Medical and surgical treatment was initially carried out by the same practitioners, but with the advent of written techniques and greater divisions in class systems, the two disciplines evolved into separate practices. In the mid to late nineteenth century, various forms of local and general anesthesia were used successfully and further facilitated the growth of modern surgery.

Surgical facilities have evolved through the centuries from the home to ultra clean, ventilated, well-lit facilities that are in use today. In 1929, Lavinia Dock wrote about early nurses preparing a private home for the arrival of a surgeon. In many cases, the kitchen table was used for an OR table and the surgeon carried the instrumentation in his black bag. Often the instruments were simply wiped clean and not washed with soap and water. Most patient preferred the privacy of their homes. Surgery was performed infrequently, and the range of procedures was limited because of high mortality.

Throughout history, hotels and monasteries in Europe frequently served as patient care facilities. In Canada, hospitals were established by French nuns in Quebec (1639) and Montreal (1642). The first recorded hospital in the United States evolved from a 1658 Dutch shelter house into Bellevue Hospital in Manhattan, followed by Blockly Hospital in Philadelphia in 1731. Unfortunately, both of these hospitals were filthy, barracks-style facilities with attendants of questionable character. The first medical school was opened in 1765, and it was under the influence of John Morgan, MD, that the practice of surgery was identified as a separate discipline from pharmacy and medicine. Although, for many years most medical doctors continued to make their own medications and perform surgery, the disciplines of general practice and surgery finally were accepted as separate aspects of patient care. During the nineteenth century, cleaner, more organized facilities were more widely available for housing the sick and mentally infirm.

Surgery was greatly affected by Lister's work on antisepsis in 1867. Antiseptic environments began to be more widely accepted in 1880 as surgeons began to develop more surgical techniques for exploring more complex anatomic regions of the body. In 1890, the practice of surgery increased enormously. Anesthetics were more widely used, and the success rate was much improved. X-rays were introduced in 1895. This facilitated earlier intervention for emergency patient care. The Mayo brothers performed 54 abdominal procedures between 1889 and 1892, but increased this to 612 by 1900. Within the next five years they performed a record 2,157 surgical procedures. As the level of surgical sophistication increased, so the number of surgical procedures performed grew.

STUDY QUESTIONS

1. Name and describe three specifically designated areas (zones) in the operating room suite.
2. What is the purpose of the preoperative holding area?
3. What should the humidity, temperature, and air exchanges per hour be in the sterile supply room?
4. What is the purpose of the substerile room? Where is it located in relation to the OR suite?
5. What is the recommended ratio of fresh air exchanges to recirculated air per hour in the OR?
6. What is the purpose of an anesthetic gas scavenger system?
7. What are HEPA filters and what are their functions?
8. The OR atmospheric environment should be maintained within a range of ___° F (___°C) and _____% humidity.
9. What is the purpose of a communication system in the OR?
10. The movement and storage of clean and sterile supplies are kept separate from contaminated items by space and traffic patterns. TRUE /FALSE.

CRITICAL THINKING ACTIVITIES

Diagram a conceptual design of an operating room suite. Identify the 3 main areas by level of sterility required for safe patient care. Ideas may include those identified in the main text or create a potentially workable schematic based on the principles of OR design. Include instrument processing areas, patient care areas, staff rooms, storage, and peripheral support areas.

SUMMARY OF CHAPTER 9

The design and function of modern surgical suites have improved the quality of care and the attainment of positive outcomes for patients. Specific layouts have significantly influenced aseptic technique and decreased infection rates.

ADDITIONAL REFERENCES

Dock LL, Stewart IM: *A short history of nursing* ed 2, New York, 1929, Knickerbocker Press.

Starr P: *The social transformation of American medicine,* New York, 1982, Basic Books, Inc.

CHAPTER 10   POTENTIAL SOURCES OF INJURY TO CAREGIVER AND PATIENT

Many environmental considerations include prevention of injuries to patients and personnel. Chapter 10 of the main text describes many environmental and occupational hazards and how to avoid them. The surgical suite has several inherent hazards infrequently found in other areas of the facility. These are physical, chemical, and biologic. These hazards are compounded when combined with long working hours and stress. The natural tendency to take short cuts when rushed to prepare the room between cases or to take unnecessary chances with hazardous exposure can result in permanent injury to patients and personnel.

LEARNING OBJECTIVES

- Identify potential environmental sources of injury to patients and personnel in the OR.
- Identify how to protect patients and personnel from injury in the OR.

COMPETENCY-BASED KNOWLEDGE

- Understand the rationale behind disaster drills.
- Understand the rationale for prevention of injury through proper use of equipment.
- Understand how and what can start and sustain a fire in the OR.
- Understand the potential effects of physical, chemical, and biologic hazards in the OR.

COMPETENCY-BASED SKILL

- Demonstrate ability to operate a fire extinguisher.
- Discuss the steps taken in the event of a fire or other internal disaster.
- Discuss methods that can be used to evacuate a patient from the OR.
- Demonstrate appropriate body mechanics for moving a patient.

CONSIDERATIONS FOR EVACUATION OF THE OR DURING INTERNAL DISASTER

Internal disasters are devastating to the entire institution. As OR caregivers, it is important to be willing to help wherever needed, but priority consideration should be given to the OR. This is particularly true if the disaster strikes during business hours. During this time, patients may be under the influence of general anesthesia, spinal or epidural, or totally immobile because of equipment or positioning devices. Table 10-1 gives a prioritized list of actions for a fire, but this list, in a modified form, applies to any disastrous event, such as explosion, earthquake, or bomb threat.

TABLE 10-1 PRIORITIZED ACTIONS IN THE EVENT OF A FIRE OR DISASTER
• Remove patients and personnel from immediate danger
• Sound the alarm to summon help
• Contain or extinguish any fire if present, as soon as possible
• Remove or disable fuel sources; turn off oxygen and piped in gases
• Evacuate the area
• Document the event
• Do not discard any materials involved with the incident

It is important not to panic if a disaster occurs or is pending. Remaining calm and level-headed will ensure better survivability of patients and personnel in the immediate area. Most ORs have manuals to instruct personnel what to do in case of fire or other disaster. It is advisable to read these ahead of time and have periodic drills for performance evaluation. Disaster drills offer the opportunity to learn by role playing without the risk of real injury. Often, experts or professional consultants, such as the Fire Chief, are present to critique the drill and offer suggestions for improvement. Many times their visit includes an inspection of the department, during which they evaluate risk factors and safety concerns.

Some considerations for planning an internal disaster protocol for the OR should include:
- Saving lives and minimizing injury to patients and personnel
- Ensuring complete evacuation of the area to avoid inadvertently leaving someone behind

Saving lives includes taking immediate action regardless of the surgical procedures in process. If the patient is under general anesthesia with an open wound, he or she still needs to be rescued. The availability of an Ambu bag and mask may facilitate airway management for the purposes of evacuation. The wound should be packed with saline soaked sponges and covered with sterile impervious drapes if possible. All piped-in gases should be stopped and disconnected for transport from the area. Movement of the patient will be contingent on the type of disaster, but may include rolling the OR table out of the area with the patient on it, moving the patient to a transport cart for evacuation, or several team members carrying the patient wrapped in blankets or sheets. Infection is a secondary concern if the patient is in peril. The protocol should include plans for emergency drugs that should be available to the anesthesia provider for the maintenance of the patient, particularly analgesics and amnesics. Because using oxygen tanks may be contraindicated, the patient will be bagged with room air. At some point, the patient may regain consciousness. There is no guarantee that the patient will survive the ordeal, but every effort should be made to save him or her.

The department should have a specified rallying point outside the building where everyone should meet for a head count after a departmental evacuation. All OR personnel, anesthesia providers, and surgeons should be made aware of this meeting place. The OR manager should try to bring a copy of the surgery schedule and staffing roster for the day to the meeting place. These documents will give an overview of which patients, staff, and doctors were in the vicinity and if anyone was possibly left behind. Personnel who may be hard to locate include transporters, stock room staff, instrument processing technicians, and those who may be at lunch or breaks. Other people who may be unaccounted for include sales representatives, residents, interns, and other students or visitors to the department. Some facilities require visitors to sign in at the control desk or at the information desk in the main lobby. If a copy of this log is available, this may be helpful in identifying others who may be inadvertently left behind.

The thought of an internal disaster is terrifying. The main emphasis of this chapter in the main text is to stress prevention, because the outcome of disaster is not usually favorable, especially in a vulnerable area such as the OR.

STUDY QUESTIONS

1. List three methods of preventing electricity hazards in the OR.
2. Identify and describe Three types of hazards in the OR.
3. What is OSHA and what does it do?
4. List several organizations/regulating bodies that govern the protection of personnel and patients in the OR.
5. List the principles of body mechanics that help in the prevention of back injuries.
6. What safety precautions can be taken to protect patients and personnel from the potential hazards of ionizing radiation?
7. A fire or explosion is the result of a combination of three factors, name them and give examples.
8. What does the mnemonic RACE stand for?
9. What are the six main areas of information supplied by the Material Safety Data Sheets (MSDS)?
10. In addition to an anesthetic gas scavenging system list other methods of controlling exposure to anesthetic waste.
11. Body substance isolation/universal precautions are essential methods of preventing cross infection. What should be done if a penetrating injury occurs or exposure to a body substance?
12. List the four key elements of a risk management program.

CRITICAL THINKING ACTIVITIES

1. Conduct a brainstorming session of hazard prevention activities that can be performed in the OR.
2. Conduct a brainstorming session of steps to be taken in a disaster. Include evacuation of patients and personnel from the area.

SUMMARY OF CHAPTER 10

Although the institution has the responsibility to provide a reasonably safe and secure workplace, the caregiver has the responsibility to utilize equipment and resources appropriately, thereby providing a safe level of care for the patient. The caregiver is also responsible for responding during an emergency, such as a fire or other internal disaster. The patient is vulnerable in the OR and trusts all of the caregivers, including the physicians, during the surgical procedure with his or her life. This is a special trust and should not be taken lightly. Prevention of injury by safe use of equipment and handling of potential hazards is a foremost priority in the plan of care.

SECTION FIVE SURGICAL ASEPSIS, INSTRUMENTATION, AND EQUIPMENT

CHAPTER 11   ATTIRE, SURGICAL SCRUB, GOWNING, GLOVING

Specialized attire for the OR supports the concept of aseptic technique. The scrub suit is considered part of OR aseptic technique and is designed to closely cover the body and prevent excess shedding of microorganisms, skin cells, and hair. When appropriately worn, the scrub suit is a protection for the wearer and the patient. The premise is that controlled laundering and storage of scrub suits reduces the possibility that microorganisms and vermin will accumulate within their fibers and be shed to the patient.

Scientific studies have shown that the surgical scrub (hand and arm washing with sufficient friction with an antiseptic solution) also reduces the risk of microbial transmission to the patient. Some antiseptics are formulated to have a cumulative antimicrobial effect. Sterile gowning and gloving by an aseptic procedure after the surgical scrub are currently the optimal method of preventing transmission of cross infection between caregiver and patient.

LEARNING OBJECTIVES

- Identify the components of appropriate OR attire.
- Identify the components of protective attire.
- Identify the sterile parameters of a surgical gown.

COMPETENCY-BASED KNOWLEDGE

- Understand the premise for the surgical hand scrub.
- Understand the premise for appropriate attire in the OR.
- Understand the premise for personal protective attire.

COMPETENCY-BASED SKILL

- Demonstrate the surgical hand scrub.
- Demonstrate the correct method of gowning and gloving.

STUDY QUESTIONS

1. What is OR attire and why is it worn?
2. List essential criteria for masks worn in the OR.
3. List several preventive measures taken to prevent cross infection from masks.
4. In which areas of the OR is it essential to wear masks?

5. Define surgical scrub and its purpose.
6. Identify the two principles of the surgical scrub that make it effective.
7. List several characteristics of an antiseptic skin scrubbing or prepping agent.
8. List two methods of performing a surgical scrub.
9. Gowns and gloves should be opened on a separate sterile field from other sterile packs.
   TRUE / FALSE
10. The closed gloving technique is used when changing a glove during a surgical procedure.
    TRUE / FALSE
11. When is the open gloving technique used?
12. Why is jewelry not worn in the OR?
13. What is the purpose of wearing shoe covers?
14. What is personal protective attire and when should it be worn?
15. List the areas of the sterile gown that when worn are NOT considered sterile.

CRITICAL THINKING ACTIVITIES

1. Define "Strike through".
2. Why is it necessary to wipe sterile gloves with a sterile damp towel after donning and before touching items on the sterile field?

SUMMARY OF CHAPTER 11

Understanding the standards and rationale for the surgical scrub and wearing special attire is an important aspect of perioperative patient care for the prevention of cross infection. The expected outcome of remaining infection-free throughout the perioperative experience is potentially attained by supporting this aspect of aseptic technique.

CHAPTER 12   ESSENTIALS OF ASEPSIS: APPLICATION OF PRINCIPLES OF ASEPTIC AND STERILE TECHNIQUES

Asepsis is the key to preventing infection in the OR. Aseptic technique is the process of remaining as clean as possible while keeping microorganisms to an irreducible minimum. Sterile technique incorporates aseptic technique, but involves maintenance of items and areas designated as being free of all living microorganisms, including spores.

LEARNING OBJECTIVES

- Identify parameters that exemplify aseptic technique.
- Identify sources of infection in the OR.
- Identify protective barriers in the OR.

COMPETENCY-BASED KNOWLEDGE

- Understand terminology associated with infection control.
- Understand the life cycle of microorganisms.
- Understand the role of sterile technique in the prevention of infection in the OR.

COMPETENCY-BASED SKILL

- Describe universal precautions in the perioperative setting.
- List the principles of sterile technique.
- Demonstrate a working knowledge of the principles of sterile technique.

STUDY QUESTIONS

1. Define sterile technique.
2. Define infection.
3. What are spores? Describe their characteristics.
4. What does the term "surgically clean" mean?
5. List the major areas on a person's body where the microbial population is greatest.
6. Every Patient in the OR is considered potentially infected. TRUE / FALSE
7. What is the purpose of an aseptic barrier?
8. List the precautions to be taken when handling sharps.
9. List the commonly used protective barriers in the OR and why they are used.
10. Critical items that are free of microorganisms, including spores, entering the body tissues underlying the skin and mucous membrane should be _____ (STERILE/ UNSTERILE). Semicritical items that have been mechanically cleaned and disinfected to reduce microorganisms and will come in contact with intact skin or mucous membranes are _____ (STERILE / UNSTERILE).
11. Unsterile persons should maintain a distance of _____ from the sterile field.

12. How should the integrity and sterility assurance of a sterile package be checked before opening it onto a sterile field?
13. The edges of a sterile package are considered _____ (STERILE / UNSTERILE) for the purpose of maintaining a margin of safety when opening a sterile pack.
14. If an item, such as the end of a suture, extends over the edge of the sterile field can it be brought back into the sterile field?

CRITICAL THINKING ACTIVITIES

1. When are the principles of sterile technique applied?
2. When is the optimum time for the sterile field to be created? Explain.
3. After a sterile bottle of solution is opened, is it acceptable to recap the bottle and save any unused contents for later use? Explain this concept.

SUMMARY OF CHAPTER 12

Sterility is an exact science. An item is either sterile or it is not. Sterile processing is covered in Chapter 13 of the main text and this resource manual.

CHAPTER 13 — STERILIZATION AND DISINFECTION

Proper processing of instruments and equipment benefits the patient and the institution. An expected outcome for the patient is decreased risk for infection. The institution has lower instrument repair and replacement costs if processing and handling are handled according to the manufacturer's recommendations.

LEARNING OBJECTIVES

- Identify key elements involved with instrument processing.
- Identify how instrument processing affects patient care.

COMPETENCY-BASED KNOWLEDGE

- Understand the difference between sterilization and disinfection.
- Understand when sterility is desired over disinfection for items used in patient care.

COMPETENCY-BASED SKILL

- Demonstrate two techniques for wrapping supplies for sterilization.
- Discuss the sterilization procedure for using chemical soak method.

STUDY QUESTIONS

1. What is the difference between sterilization and disinfection?
2. List three methods of sterilization.
3. Describe the procedure for proper loading of a gravity displacement steam sterilizer.
4. Biologic monitoring requires a processed, incubated indicator and an unprocessed control indicator. Explain why.
5. List the processing factors a chemical indicator can detect.
6. Discuss the recommended practice for sterilization of rubber goods.
7. How does a warm package get contaminated when it is placed on a solid, cold surface?
8. Describe the sterilization method and packaging method of choice for talc.
9. Sterilization dates are recorded on the package for what purpose?
10. What is the key factor in the determination of shelf life of a sterile item?

MATCHING EXERCISE

Place the number of the recommended processing level of the instrument or equipment for safe patient use.

LEVEL OF PROCESSING	INSTRUMENT OR EQUIPMENT USED IN PATIENT CARE
11. Critical (Sterile) 12. Semicritical (Disinfected) 13. Noncritical (Unsterile)	___hysteroscope ___implant ___airway ___blood pressure cuff ___suction tip ___hemostat ___stethoscope ___bronchoscope ___biopsy forceps ___cystoscope

CRITICAL THINKING ACTIVITIES

Write a paragraph describing the sequence of events in a gravity displacement steam sterilizer. How does this differ in a prevacuum sterilizer?

SUMMARY OF CHAPTER 13

Sterilization and disinfection are important aspects of patient care in the OR. Standards should be followed for each processing method to ensure the highest quality of instrument and equipment preparation. Prevention of infection and injury decreases the risk of wasting scarce resources. Instrumentation will remain in good condition and fewer repairs and/or replacements will be needed. The result will be a better blend of controlled health care costs and better attainment of expected outcomes.

CHAPTER 14 — SURGICAL INSTRUMENTATION

Surgical instrumentation is critical for the performance of the surgical procedure. Knowing each instrument by name, how it is handled and processed, and how it is used will increase the efficiency of the OR team. The surgical procedure will proceed smoothly and expected outcomes will be attained if the instrumentation is correctly processed and used.

LEARNING OBJECTIVES

- Identify several types of dissecting instruments.
- Identify several types of grasping instruments.
- Distinguish between crushing and noncrushing clamps.
- Identify several items on the sterile field that are considered to be "sharps".

COMPETENCY-BASED KNOWLEDGE

- Understand how proper placement of an instrument in someone's hand facilitates its use.
- Understand the rationale for decontaminating all items on the sterile field after a procedure.
- Understand the rationale for the methods used in assembly of instrument sets.

COMPETENCY-BASED SKILL

- Demonstrate the correct method of passing an instrument to another person's hand.
- Demonstrate several methods of passing sharps to the field.
- Demonstrate how to assemble and check power equipment.

STUDY QUESTIONS

1. Name several causes of surgical instrumentation corrosion.
2. Match the instrument to the appropriate classification:

   A. Dissecting   ____ Allis forceps
   B. Grasping   ____ Scissors
   C. Occluding   ____ Rake
   D. Exposing   ____ Hemostat

3. Match the scalpel blade number with its description:

   A   #10   ____ Straight edge with pointed tip
   B   #11   ____ Medium round cutting edge
   C   #12   ____ Large round cutting edge
   D   #15   ____ Hook-like, cutting edge on inside curve
   E   #20   ____ Small, short, round cutting edge

4. Match the following suction tips to the appropriate application:
   a. Poole   ___ Mouth
   b. Frazier   ___ Abdominal cavity
   c. Yankauer   ___ Used when little or no fluid, except capillary bleeding
   d. Aspirating tube ___ Through the endoscope
5. What is the use of a probe?
6. Identify two safety precautions used with power equipment.
7. How should instruments be inspected before packaging them for use?
8. Describe the assembly of an instrument set for sterilization.

CRITICAL THINKING ACTIVITIES

Contact several instrument sales representatives for catalogs of surgical instruments. Some manufacturers have incorporated modifications or design enhancements that differ from illustrations included in the main text. Some surgical specialties use angled or longer versions of standard instruments. Some vascular clamps and scissors are classified as left- and right-handed according to the curve of the tip.

SUMMARY OF CHAPTER 14

Many varieties of instruments are available through many different companies. Some are geared for a particular specialty; others are more generic and multipurpose. The key element is in the proper care and handling to make them efficient and safe for use in the care of the patient.

CHAPTER 15 — SPECIALIZED SURGICAL EQUIPMENT

Technologic advances foster the development of more complex equipment and machinery for use in patient care. Perioperative nurses and surgical technologists have the responsibility to remain current in their knowledge of new techniques and procedures that require specialized equipment and machines. Personnel and patients are placed at risk for injury when new technologies are not used under safe conditions.

LEARNING OBJECTIVES

- Identify several types of lasers used in the OR.
- Distinguish between monopolar and bipolar electrosurgical unit use.
- Identify several types of endoscopic equipment.

COMPETENCY-BASED KNOWLEDGE

- Understand how different lasers have different tissue effects in vivo.
- Understand how electric current affects tissue.
- Understand the hazards of tissue plume in the OR.
- Understand safety factors associated with the use of electrosurgical units.
- Understand safety factors associated with the use of lasers.
- Understand the advantages and disadvantages of specialized equipment in surgery.

COMPETENCY-BASED SKILL

- Demonstrate how lasers are tested before the patient is brought into the room.
- Discuss how endoscopy, lasers, and electrosurgical units can be used in combination for the same surgical procedure.

STUDY QUESTIONS

1. Explain why electrosurgery is not used for the initial incision.
2. Explain why a dispersive electrode is not needed with bipolar electrosurgery.
3. Where is the safest location for placement of the dispersive electrode for the patient who had a total hip prosthesis implanted 15 years ago in his right side?
4. Electrosurgery should not be used in the mouth, around the head, or in the pleural cavity when high concentrations of _____ are present.
5. Documentation of electrosurgical unit use in the OR includes:
6. A CO_2 insufflator is used to create a pneumoperitoneum to allow for visualization of organs and structures within the peritoneal cavity. The safe CO_2 flow pressure range is maintained between _____ mm Hg.
7. Laser safety glasses or goggles of the correct optical density are worn at all times while the laser is in use. TRUE / FALSE

8. Contact lenses are adequate eye protection for CO_2 laser. TRUE / FALSE
9. When lens covers with filter caps are used during a laser microscopic case, the rest of the surgical team does not need to wear individual eye protection. TRUE / FALSE
10. When the CO_2 laser is used moistened sponges or towels are placed around the targeted tissue to protect the area from thermal injury. TRUE / FALSE
11. The rectum should be packed with a moistened sponge to prevent methane gas from escaping from the intestinal tract during use of the CO_2 laser in the perineal area. TRUE / FALSE
12. Laser and Bovie plume contains toxic substances that may become airborne from vaporization of tissues. TRUE / FALSE
13. Gloves, eyewear, and mask are worn when changing smoke evacuator filters. TRUE / FALSE

CRITICAL THINKING ACTIVITIES

1. Discuss the effects of overdistending the patient's abdomen during an abdominal laparoscopic procedure.
2. Discuss the pros and cons of endoscopic, minimally invasive procedures.

SUMMARY OF CHAPTER 15

Specialized surgical equipment is safe and effective for patient care when operated by trained users, maintained as per manufacturer's recommendations, and used appropriately for its intended purpose.

SECTION SIX: PREOPERATIVE PATIENT CARE

CHAPTER 16 — PREOPERATIVE PREPARATION OF THE PATIENT

The circulator may not have the opportunity to interview or assess the patient preoperatively. A head-to-toe assessment or review of systems approach may not be practical. During the identification procedure, the circulator is responsible for checking data documented by others. The emphasis of this chapter is on communication between all caregivers, the patient, and the patient's family and/or significant others.

LEARNING OBJECTIVES

- Understand the importance of preoperative caregiver-patient communication.
- Understand how psychologic preparation of the patient affects outcomes.

COMPETENCY-BASED KNOWLEDGE

- Discuss the content of preoperative teaching.
- Describe empathic awareness of the patient's needs by OR personnel.

COMPETENCY-BASED SKILL

- Demonstrate communication techniques that apply to all patients and significant others.
- Demonstrate communication techniques that apply to special needs patients.

STUDY QUESTIONS

1. Name several techniques taught to patients preoperatively that can reduce postoperative complications.
2. What is the purpose of the perioperative nurse's preoperative assessment?
3. Describe the style of interview questions that allow the patient to respond freely, sharing feelings and concerns.
4. A good time to conduct an interview and instruct the patient is the morning of surgery. TRUE / FALSE
5. List several tips to remember when interviewing a patient.
6. The perioperative nurse should not discuss the operating suite and the routines since the patient will have postoperative amnesia caused by medication and anesthesia. TRUE / FALSE
7. The perioperative nurse should encourage the patient to discuss feelings and anxiety. TRUE / FALSE
8. Discuss some special needs identified in the preoperative assessment that assist the OR team during the implementation phase of the plan of care.

9. Name three levels of preoperative teaching.
10. Why should the family and/or significant other be included in preoperative teaching?
11. Why is it necessary for the anesthesia provider to assess the patient preoperatively?
12. A preoperative check list is completed to ensure the patient is properly prepared for the surgical procedure. Name several items that should be included on the check list.
13. Upon the arrival of the patient to the OR, the circulator should check for which items on the patient's chart?
14. List the role of the circulator during induction of anesthesia.
15. Preoperative preparation can influence the outcome of the surgical procedure. TRUE / FALSE

Pros and Cons of preoperative visits by perioperative nurse. Place a P or C in the space provided to denote whether the item is Pro or Con.	P or C
1. Experienced interviewer educates and prepares the patient and family for OR	1. ____
2. Improve intraoperative patient care and efficiency	2. ____
3. Cost increase for adequate staffing	3. ____
4. Foster meaningful nurse-patient-significant other relationships	4. ____
5. Timing is difficult with same day admissions	5. ____
6. OR staff may not be skilled in making visits	6. ____
7. Promotes patient cooperation and involvement by facilitating communication	7. ____
8. Contributes to positive self-image of the caregiver	8. ____
9. Repetitive questioning can lead to lack of enthusiasm and spontaneity	9. ____
10. Interviewer may have personal biases that can influence objectivity	10. ____

CRITICAL THINKING ACTIVITIES

Role-play scenarios help caregivers to develop communication skills. Plan learning scenarios between two learners to include playing the role of the patient and the interviewer. Changing the scenario to include good and bad interviewing techniques may help illustrate the most therapeutic communication skills to develop. Reversing roles also helps to demonstrate the subjective effects of the communication process. Suggested role playing exercises include, but are not limited to:

- Caregiver and Pediatric patient's parents
- Caregiver and Pediatric patient
- Caregiver and Hearing impaired geriatric patient
- Caregiver and Non English speaking patient
- Caregiver and Cooperative patient
- Caregiver and Uncooperative patient
- Caregiver and Adolescent patient in presence of parents
- Caregiver and Patient having a palliative procedure for terminal illness

SUMMARY OF CHAPTER 16

Communication between the patient, significant others, and caregiver is important in preoperative psychologic preparation. The more prepared the patient is the higher degree of cooperation may be elicited. Including the patient's significant others in preoperative planning helps to establish baselines for evaluating the attainment of expected outcomes throughout the perioperative experience.

Communication between caregivers is essential for the implementation phase of the nursing process. Preoperative caregivers should make sure the chart is complete before the patient goes to the OR. When time precludes the possibility of a perioperative nurse visiting the patient preoperatively, some of the most salient assessment factors are derived from the documentation of other caregivers. Incomplete or inaccurate data is a potential source of injury to the patient. If a preoperative interview by the perioperative nurse is not possible, the following factors should be assessed before placing the patient on the OR table, and most certainly before the induction of anesthesia according to established institutional policy and procedure:

- confirmed identity of the patient
- confirmation of the intended surgical procedure, surgeon, and informed consent
- type of anesthesia to be used
- allergies and comorbid conditions (i.e., diabetes, cardiac disease, current medications)
- special instrumentation, equipment, and supplies needed (i.e., implant or prosthesis availability)
- special positioning or prepping needs
- presence and location of family and/or significant others

SECTION SEVEN: ANESTHESIA CONCEPTS AND CONSIDERATIONS

CHAPTER 17   GENERAL ANESTHESIA: TECHNIQUES AND AGENTS

The patient is very vulnerable during the intraoperative phase of care. This is because the patient may be receiving medications or other consciousness altering substances that can impair cognition and reasoning. When the plan of care includes the administration of general anesthesia the level of vulnerability increases immensely. Under general anesthesia, the patient becomes totally unconscious and totally dependent on the OR team. Chapter 17 of the main text explores the history, administration, and implications of general anesthesia.

LEARNING OBJECTIVES

- Identify three methods for administration of general anesthesia.
- Identify measures to encourage the patient's feeling of security.

COMPETENCY-BASED KNOWLEDGE

- Understand rationale behind the selection of anesthetic agents.
- Understand the physiologic effects of general anesthesia.
- Understand the hazards of general anesthesia.

COMPETENCY-BASED SKILL

- Demonstrate cricoid pressure.
- Demonstrate several methods of safe patient handling during general anesthesia.

STUDY QUESTIONS

1. What is the purpose of cricoid pressure (Sellick's maneuver)?
2. Name the neuromuscular blocker used primarily for endotracheal intubation.
3. Endogenous endorphins in the body bind to opiate receptors in the brain and spinal cord. TRUE / FALSE
4. List three methods of administration of general anesthesia.
5. Pain is purely organic. TRUE / FALSE
6. The lessening of or insensitivity to pain is _____.
7. Considerations in the choice of anesthetic agents should include:
8. List the purposes of muscle relaxants (neuromuscular blockers).
9. Intraoperative awareness (auditory stimuli) varies depending on the depth of anesthesia. List the sounds that the patient may remember after emergence from general anesthesia.
10. Discuss 5 main objectives in the maintenance of general anesthesia.

MATCHING: Each letter or term is used only once.

A	B
1. Antimuscarinic	_____ Midazolam (Versed)
2. Neuromuscular blocker	_____ Narcotics (Opiate)
3. Amnesics	_____ Hydroxyzine hydrochloride (Vistaril)
4. Analgesic	_____ Atropine sulfate
5. IV Conscious Sedation	_____ Propofol (Diprivan)
6. Antiemetic	_____ Sedatives and tranquilizers
7. Anesthetic	_____ Atracurium besylate (Tracrium)

CRITICAL THINKING ACTIVITIES

Develop group scenarios depicting dependent situations. Suggested group activities for the learning lab include:

Patient Simulation
- Simulate an unconscious patient lying on an OR table. Have several learners (preferably 4) take turns changing the sample patient's position, taking into consideration the patient's helplessness. Put the sample patient's limbs through normal range of motion. Using appropriate body mechanics, the group could reposition the sample patient from supine, to lateral, to prone, and then back to supine. After the exercise, conduct a group discussion about the group dynamics needed to care for a patient who is under general anesthesia. The learner, who played the role of the patient, should also describe the experience. Each participant should have the opportunity to play the patient.

Free Fall
- This scenario is designed to depict the confidence the patient has in the caregiver. Several learners (preferably 4) can stand in a row closely behind a simulated patient who is blindfolded. On the count of three the simulated patient falls backward into the waiting arms of the other learners. Discussions after this exercise should include how it felt to be responsible for catching the simulated patient. The simulated patient should recount how he or she felt during the fall. Each participant should have the opportunity to try the free fall. Discussion should be based on the balance of responsibility for the well-being of another person and the dependency of the patient. This exercise exemplifies the concept of trust.

SUMMARY CHAPTER 17

The OR team has the responsibility to protect the patient at all times throughout the intraoperative period. The environment should be safe and the patient should feel secure. Many hazards are inherent to the administration of anesthesia. The plan of care for the use of general anesthesia should be personalized for the needs of each patient, based on physiologic and psychologic assessment data.

CHAPTER 18   LOCAL AND REGIONAL ANESTHESIA

Caring for a conscious patient who is having a surgical procedure under local anesthesia requires additional consideration for psychologic and physiologic factors. Psychologic issues include the ongoing sights and sounds of the OR in process, such as instrumentation in use or talk of the OR team. Physiologically, the patient is conscious and not dependent on ventilatory support or other supplementary homeostatic agent. It is important to monitor for physiologic changes throughout the procedure because agents used for local and regional anesthesia can cause an unexpected reaction in a susceptible patient. During local anesthesia, the patient should be monitored by a qualified perioperative nurse who can institute resuscitative measures as needed. During regional and MAC procedures, an anesthesia provider should be present and monitoring the patient at all times.

LEARNING OBJECTIVES

- Differentiate between local and regional anesthesia.
- Differentiate between an expected response and an untoward response to anesthesia.

COMPETENCY-BASED KNOWLEDGE

- Understand the mechanism behind altered sensory perception at nerve endings after the administration of a local anesthetic.
- Identify several sensory nerve endings in the body and discuss their functions.
- Discuss the psychologic impact of sights and sounds in the OR on the patient receiving local anesthesia.

COMPETENCY-BASED SKILL

- Demonstrate the use and interpretation of monitoring equipment used during the administration of local anesthesia.
- Prepare the OR environment for a patient who will be receiving local anesthesia.
- Simulate resuscitation of the patient who has had an adverse reaction to local anesthesia.

STUDY QUESTIONS

1. Describe the action and benefits of local anesthesia.
2. Describe patient care during the use of local anesthesia.
3. List several advantages of local anesthesia.
4. List several disadvantages of local anesthesia.
5. List the effects of IV conscious sedation.
6. List several patient responses to observe for when monitoring the patient receiving local anesthesia.
7. List the features of regional blocks.

8. In monitored anesthesia care (MAC), an anesthesia provider is present. TRUE / FALSE
9. An advantage of local anesthesia is that a surgeon can administer the anesthetic in the absence of an anesthesia provider. TRUE / FALSE
10. Spinal headaches are caused by persistent cerebrospinal fluid leaking through the dura. TRUE / FALSE

CRITICAL THINKING ACTIVITIES

1. Local and regional anesthesia specifically diminish sensory interpretation by nerve endings in the area of application. In some areas of the body, pain perception may be dulled, but touch and temperature sensation are still perceived. Consider how sensory mechanisms work in various areas of the body and identify nerve endings that may respond to anesthetic agents. Table 18-1 lists sensory neurons located throughout various areas of the body.
2. Discuss how different areas of the body use end organs or nerve endings for interpretation of sensory stimuli.

TABLE 18-1

Sensory neurons: contained in the end organs (body and organ surfaces) in the peripheral nervous system (PNS)
- Exteroceptors - external body surface, respond to superficial stimuli, such as to skin or mucous membrane: sense touch, temperature, pain, and sound vibration
- Interoceptors / visceroceptors - found in organs and respond to stimuli within the viscera, such as digestion, excretion, or blood pressure
- Proprioceptors - found in muscles, tendons, joints, and vestibule of inner ear: responds to body locomotion, equilibrium, spatial orientation, and posture
- Mechanocreceptors - found throughout the body: respond to muscular contractions, pressure, stretch, sound, touch, and sound vibration
- Thermoreceptors - sensory endings specifically sensitive to temperature change
- Photoreceptors - found in retina: respond to light stimuli
- Chemoreceptors - found in carotid arteries: respond to chemical change in blood stimulates the respiratory center, such as elevated blood CO_2 level
- Nociceptors - somatic and visceral nerve endings, thinly myelinated or unmyelinated nerves, respond to endogenous chemical stimuli and inflammation: injury sensors

SUMMARY OF CHAPTER 18

The application of local or regional anesthesia is intended to cause decreased sensory interpretation in a specific area of the body. The patient is usually still aware of the environment on a conscious level and should be considered in the plan of care. Monitoring for untoward responses, either physiologic or psychologic, should be a team effort but primarily performed by a qualified perioperative nurse in the absence of an anesthesia provider. Appropriate monitoring equipment and safeguards should be employed at all times while the patient is in the care of perioperative caregivers.

CHAPTER 19 PATIENT MONITORING AND POTENTIAL COMPLICATIONS RELATED TO ANESTHESIA

Regardless of the surgical procedure and the type of anesthesia employed, the patient requires physiologic monitoring throughout the entire perioperative care period. Preoperatively, baselines are determined and compared to periodic checking intervals intraoperatively and postoperatively. Without baselines, subsequent monitoring may not reveal progressive deviation from normal physiologic parameters. Initial measurements should be taken before any interventions have taken place. Stress and physical manipulation can cause false readings. Caregivers should observe the patient in comparison with any monitoring devices because a miscalibration could lead to an inaccurate readout on a machine. The expected outcome of monitoring should reflect the desire to detect an abnormality and effect corrective action immediately. Without pre-, intra-, and postoperative monitoring, a physiologic problem may go unnoticed until it is advanced. Simple corrections may include administration of O_2 or increasing the flow rate of the IV. More complex interventions may include administration of medication or full life support. Prevention of extremes provides for the best outcome for the patient.

LEARNING OBJECTIVES

- Identify several body systems that should be monitored during a surgical procedure.
- Differentiate between invasive and noninvasive monitoring equipment and devices.

COMPETENCY-BASED KNOWLEDGE

- Understand the interrelationships between body systems and how this reflects the patient's homeostasis.
- Understand why patient monitoring and interpretation of monitoring data are equally important.

COMPETENCY-BASED SKILL

- Demonstrate how several noninvasive monitors are applied to the patient.
- Demonstrate skill in interpreting data derived from noninvasive monitoring equipment.

STUDY QUESTIONS

1. List several key issues involving the use of monitoring equipment.
2. What are the differences between invasive and noninvasive patient monitoring?
3. List the complications of intravascular hemodynamic monitoring.
4. List several sites for intravascular cannulation.
5. Is an ECG tracing on the monitor visible during asystole?
6. Describe sinus rhythm as it appears on the cardiac monitor.
7. How is urinary output compared to cardiac function?

8. What is the difference between peripheral cyanosis and central cyanosis?
9. What information does temperature monitoring provide.
10. List two neurologic monitors used during surgery
11. List several complications that can affect the patient under anesthesia.
12. List several methods of drug administration in the OR.

CRITICAL THINKING ACTIVITIES

What information about the patient's condition should the caregiver expect to identify during noninvasive monitoring of a patient? Exercise 19-2 (page 57) is designed to simulate monitoring by several noninvasive methods. Interpretation of assessment data is critical in the prevention of undesired outcomes. For example, the initial assessment may reveal tachycardia that in the later stages of a serious condition becomes bradycardia. This progression may be shown in the exercise as I_J. Some problematic conditions may show all of the assessment parameters as the onset progresses from initial stages to a full life threatening crisis. A separate sheet of paper may be needed to accommodate the volume of data for each possible patient condition.

SUMMARY OF CHAPTER 19

The importance of patient monitoring and interpretation of assessment data obtained from monitoring is key to the well-being of the patient. All of the monitors known to modern medical science have no meaning if the person using them cannot interpret the data. Knowledge and skill applied to patient monitoring can be helpful in the early recognition of a potentially lethal patient condition. Early treatment of a potential problem offers the best chance for a favorable patient outcome.

EXERCISE 19-2 Each letter is used multiple times. List **ALL** letters as they apply.

NONINVASIVE MONITORING		INTERPRETATION OF ADULT ASSESSMENT DATA		POSSIBLE PATIENT CONDITION
Respirations	A	rapid, labored	rate above 22, using accessory muscles	ANXIETY
	B	shallow, slow	rate below 14, little chest excursion	
	C	even, easy	rate between 16-20 per minute	
Skin	A	cool, dry	pale, pink	METABOLIC EVENT
	B	cool, moist	pale	
	C	hot	may be flushed or ruddy	
	D	mottled	cyanosis, duskiness	
	E	diaphoresis	wet, sweating	
Blood pressure	A	hypotension	diastolic pressure ↓ 60 mm Hg	MALIGNANT HYPERTHERMIA
	B	hypertension	systolic pressure ↑ 130 mm Hg	
	C	normotension	systolic 100-120; diastolic 70-80 mm Hg	
Pulse rate	A	bradycardia	rate below 60 per minute	HYPOTHERMIA
	B	tachycardia	rate over 100 per minute	
	C	normal	between 72-90 per minute	
Pulse rhythm	A	full	easy to palpate	HYPOVOLEMIA
	B	thready	weak, difficult to palpate	
	C	full and bounding	very forceful and extreme	
Electrocardiogram	A	regular sinus rhythm	P wave precedes each QRS complex	HYPOXEMIA
	B	premature atrial beats	P waves without a QRS complex	
	C	premature ventricular beats	QRS complexes without P waves	
Pulse oximeter	A	O_2 reading below 90%	central cyanosis, duskiness of lips	HYPERVOLEMIA
	B	O_2 reading above 90%	peripheral cyanosis, bluish nail beds	
	C	O_2 reading of 97-100%	skin pink, no signs of cyanosis	
Temperature	A	hypothermia	core temperature below 96°F (35°C)	DRUG INTERACTION
	B	hyperthermia	core temperature above 100.4°F (38°C)	
	C	normothermia	core temperature 98.2°-99.9°F (36.8°-37.7°C)	
Consciousness	A	awake	alert and cognizant of surroundings	SHOCK
	B	drowsiness	rouses to cognizance	
	C	confusion	rouses, but not cognizant of surroundings	
	D	unconscious	not rousable	

SECTION EIGHT: INTRAOPERATIVE PATIENT CARE

CHAPTER 20 — COORDINATED ROLES OF SCRUB PERSON AND CIRCULATOR

Caring for the perioperative patient is a concerted effort of the entire OR team. The coordination of roles between the scrub person and the circulator keeps the surgical procedure on an even pace while maintaining the separation between sterile and unsterile aspects of the patient's care.

LEARNING OBJECTIVES

- Identify common preliminary preparatory tasks of the scrub and circulator.
- Identify preparatory tasks of the scrub person.
- Identify preparatory tasks of the circulator.

COMPETENCY-BASED KNOWLEDGE

- Understand the implication of specific roles in regard to educational preparation of each team member.
- Understand the rationale for setting up the sterile field as close to the time of the procedure as possible.
- Understand the rationale for disassembly and complete processing of sets if a case is opened, then canceled.

COMPETENCY-BASED SKILL

- Demonstrate the preliminary preparation of the OR for the first patient of the day.
- Demonstrate the creation and maintenance of a sterile field.
- Demonstrate opening sterile packs and placing the contents on the sterile field.
- Demonstrate correct manner of passing instruments between sterile team members.
- Demonstrate acceptable methods of transferring sterile, unwrapped items from the autoclave to the sterile field.
- Demonstrate acceptable methods of counting and accounting for all items on the sterile field.

STUDY QUESTIONS

1. When packs or sets have been wrapped with double wrappers, the outer wrap is considered the _____ and the inner wrap is considered the _____.
2. Who opens which layer of a double-wrapped pack or set?
3. If a sterile package wrapped in woven materials is dropped to the floor can it still be transferred to the sterile field? Why?
4. How is shelf life determined?

5. Describe the method of draping a nonsterile table.
6. Who is responsible for counting sponges, sharps, and instruments in surgery?
7. What precautions should be taken when a solution or medication is dispensed onto the sterile field to prevent a medication error?
8. At what temperature should irrigation solution be used?

To maintain sterility, the entire team should watch for any breaks in sterile technique and remedy them immediately. Questions 9 - 12 give specific incidents wherein the integrity of the sterile field is interrupted. List the corrective actions.

9. A sterile team member contaminates a glove, gown, or sleeve.
10. A sterile team member's glove is perforated by a needle or torn by an instrument, the skin is not broken.
11. A sterile team member needs to change places with another sterile team member.
12. Why should the table remain intact and the setup remain sterile until the patient has left the room?
13. Where is the optimal place to position the dispersive electrode for use with a monopolar electrosurgical unit?
14. List several main points of preparing a specimen for the laboratory.
15. What is the purpose of a counting procedure for sponges, sharps, and instruments?

CRITICAL THINKING ACTIVITIES

1. Write a narrative describing the responsibilities of the circulator during the surgical procedure up to and including wound closure.
2. List the steps to be taken by the scrub person and circulator when there is an incorrect count.
3. Write a narrative describing the information that should be documented by the circulator on the patient's OR record during the intraoperative phase of care.
4. What are the responsibilities of the circulator while the anesthesia provider is beginning the induction of anesthesia?.

SUMMARY OF CHAPTER 20

Each member of the team has a specific role in the care of the patient. Before, during, and after the procedure, observance of sterile technique and aseptic practices supports the attainment of expected outcomes for the patient. Primarily, the scrub person is concerned with the technical aspects of the procedure, such as the set up, flow of the case from the sterile perspective, and the tear down of the set up after the patient leaves the room. The circulator, on the other hand, is concerned with the total flow of the procedure and the needs of the patient, the OR team, and the anesthesia provider. The circulator is the main communication link between the OR and the patient's family and/or significant others. Subsequent procedures scheduled to follow are dependent on information provided by the circulator concerning the flow of the case in process. If the current case is running over or finishing early, the timing of the next scheduled procedure may need to be moved to another room or moved up in time.

CHAPTER 21 — POSITIONING THE PATIENT

Positioning the patient for the surgical procedure is as critical to the well-being of the patient as the procedure itself. The intent of the positioning process is to provide exposure of the surgical site. The physical act of positioning the patient should not injure joints, muscles, tendons, ligaments, nerves, or soft tissue. The motions should be smooth, precise, and gently performed. Extreme ranges of motion may cause stretch damage to nerves or ligaments. Maintenance of the position should be accomplished by sturdy, but tissue sparing devices, such as well-padded table attachments. No part of the patient should be at jeopardy for damage from prolonged pressure against a hard surface. Individual physical differences should be incorporated in the positioning plan and modifications to the positioning procedure should be made. Height, weight, physical stature, missing limbs, or other anatomic anomalies may affect how the patient is placed and maintained in a modified form of a standardized position. For example, the lithotomy position would need to be modified for a unilateral or bilateral lower extremity amputee.

Other considerations include the use of commercial warming devices, such as hypo-, hyperthermia blankets or forced air warming systems. Substantial injury could occur from excess heat in the form of burns. Consider also that extreme temperatures may increase metabolism and cause the patient to lose body fluids through perspiration.

Postoperative evaluation of the expected outcomes related to the positioning process should include physical inspection of the patient's body surfaces for signs of discoloration, abrasion, or other surface injury. It is also important to investigate any complaints of numbness, tingling, or paresthesia. Any limb that has been used for vascular access or for automatic blood pressure readings is at risk, as well as any limb that was part of the surgical site. Most complaints about limb discomfort associated with the surgical site should normalize within a reasonable length of time during the postanesthesia recovery period. All complaints should be investigated by a physician. Documentation of the patient's specific statements may lead to discovery of the cause of the discomfort. The expected outcome is that the patient will be free of untoward sequelae caused by positioning from the surgical procedure.

LEARNING OBJECTIVES

- Identify potential safety hazards associated with moving a patient from one surface to another.
- Identify anatomic considerations associated with positioning.
- Identify positioning aids, equipment, and table attachments used in patient positioning.

COMPETENCY-BASED KNOWLEDGE

- Understand how positioning affects the patient's major body systems.
- Understand how appropriate positioning facilitates the surgical procedure.

COMPETENCY-BASED SKILL

- Demonstrate several safe methods of transferring the patient from a transport vehicle to the OR table.
- Demonstrate the procedure for placing the patient into a lateral position.
- Demonstrate the procedure for placing the patient into a prone position.
- Demonstrate the procedure for placing the patient into a lithotomy position.

STUDY QUESTIONS

1. Proper positioning of the patient during surgery includes:
2. What determines the position that the patient will be positioned in?
3. What physiologic factors influence patient positioning?
4. Who has joint responsibility for placing the patient in the correct surgical position?
5. What factors influence the timing of patient positioning?
6. List the safety measures that should be observed while transferring the patient from the transport cart to the OR table.
7. What positioning aids relieve pressure on the anterior thorax and facilitate chest expansion when a patient is in the prone position?
8. Name 5 major body systems taken into consideration during positioning for a surgical procedure.
9. Identify the surgical positions that would limit motion of the chest for respiration. What can be done to decrease this limitation?
10. When placing a patient in the lithotomy position, why is it important to raise both legs simultaneously?

CRITICAL THINKING ACTIVITIES

Create a list including each major body system. For each system, identify two surgical procedures that require separate positions. Diagram the positions, complete with incision lines. For each illustration, identify and list the main body systems affected by each position.

SUMMARY OF CHAPTER 21

Anatomic considerations of safe and comfortable patient positioning include preventing compromise of body systems, providing exposure of the surgical site, maintaining access for anesthesia administration, and preventing patient injury.

CHAPTER 22	SKIN PREPARATION AND DRAPING OF THE SURGICAL SITE

The outcome of the surgical procedure is in part influenced by the manner in which the patient is psychologically and physiologically prepared. Psychologic preparation is discussed in Chapter 16 of the main text and this resource manual. This initial component of the preparation process helps the patient make decisions about treatment options and allows him or her to contribute to the plan of care. Physiologic preparation is performed in two main stages. The first stage is the preoperative assessment and/or testing. This leads to any remedial or prophylactic systemic pharmacologic therapy needed for homeostatic support before surgery. The second stage is when the patient enters the OR. The patient is positioned and the actual surgical site is locally prepared with antiseptic solution and draped using sterile technique. Proper positioning and draping facilitates the performance of the procedure. Skin cleansing and maintaining sterile conditions helps to protect the patient from infection. Inadequate total preparation for the intended surgical procedure could leave the patient vulnerable to undesired outcomes both psychologically and physiologically.

LEARNING OBJECTIVES

- Identify keys elements involved with physiologic preparation of the patient.
- Identify potential problems that can be anticipated if the physiologic preparation of the patient is inadequate.

COMPETENCY-BASED KNOWLEDGE

- Understand the chemical and mechanical actions of the skin preparation procedure.
- Understand the principles of the draping procedure.

COMPETENCY-BASED SKILL

- Demonstrate the skin preparation procedure.
- Demonstrate the use of sterile technique in a patient draping procedure.

STUDY QUESTIONS

1. What is the purpose of preoperative skin preparation?
2. When is the most appropriate time for hair removal for a surgical procedure?
3. Name two areas of the body where depilatory creams are not used for hair removal.
4. The antiseptic agent used for skin preparation should have certain qualities. List these qualities.
5. Drapes should be porous to prevent heat buildup and maintain an isothermic environment appropriate for the patient's body temperature. TRUE / FALSE
6. Why should drapes be lint free and antistatic?

7. What are the advantages of a self-adhering plastic drape?
8. What is a thermal drape made of and what does it do?
9. If a sterile drape has been incorrectly positioned, it can be readjusted to the correct position. TRUE / FALSE
10. Describe the desirable qualities of draping material.

CRITICAL THINKING ACTIVITIES

Write a narrative describing the process of preparing the patient's skin for a surgical procedure.
- Discuss preparation procedures for hair removal, such as shaving, clipping of hair, and the use of depilatories. Discuss the different types of solutions that can be used for skin preparation and why one solution may be chosen over another. Include a discussion of why a patient who is allergic to iodine or shell fish should not be prepped with an iodine-based solution.
- Discuss the implication of local versus systemic allergy to iodine.
- Describe how the areas that will remain contaminated within the surgical field are prepped, such as stomas and body orifices.

SUMMARY OF CHAPTER 22

Physical preparation of the patient may include inserting an indwelling Foley catheter, positioning, hair removal, antiseptic cleansing of the surgical site, and draping for exposure. One expected outcome of the surgical procedure is to be free of infection. These procedures are performed under strict sterile conditions to prevent contamination of the surgical site for the best outcome for the patient.

CHAPTER 23   HEMOSTASIS AND BLOOD LOSS REPLACEMENT

Blood is vital to life. Hemostasis is the process by which bleeding is controlled. Common ways to control bleeding include chemical, mechanical, and thermal methods. The advent of transfusions, both autologous and homologous, give the hemorrhaging patient another chance at life when blood loss is uncontrollable and other means of hemostasis have failed.

Estimation of blood loss includes observing amounts in suction canisters, visual inspection of field and drapes, and actual bloody sponge weight. Visual observation and estimation of blood loss is generally acceptable for most procedures, but pediatric and compromised patients' sponges should be weighed for accuracy. Irrigation and body fluids, such as urine or ascitic fluid should be accounted for in the volume loss calculation.

LEARNING OBJECTIVES

- Identify several chemical methods of hemostasis.
- Identify several mechanical methods of hemostasis.
- Identify several thermal methods of hemostasis.

COMPETENCY-BASED KNOWLEDGE

- Understand the physiologic basis for the blood clotting mechanism.
- Understand the potential for injury during alteration or occlusion of blood flow to a body part.

COMPETENCY-BASED SKILL

- Demonstrate safe and effective practices when using chemical methods of hemostasis.
- Demonstrate safe and effective practices when using mechanical methods of hemostasis.
- Demonstrate the procedure for weighing sponges for blood loss estimate.
- Demonstrate safe and effective practices when using thermal methods of hemostasis.

STUDY QUESTIONS

1. List the steps in the natural process of hemostasis.
2. When using a sequential pneumatic compression device, what information should the circulator document on the intraoperative record?
3. What is the primary purpose for a pneumatic counter pressure device?
4. What are some of the precautions the circulator should be aware of when using the pneumatic tourniquet?
5. Name 3 stressors that can precipitate a sickle cell crisis.
6. What assessment data would the circulator need to care for a patient with hemophilia?
7. What is the most desired source of blood for transfusion?

8. How can postoperative deep vein thrombosis be prevented?
9. A postoperative patient is complaining of pain at the surgical site and is hypotensive, tachycardiac, restless, thirsty, and appears pale. The perioperative nurse should assess the patient for what possible complication?
10. Surgical removal is the only way to treat pulmonary emboli. TRUE / FALSE

MATCHING: HEMOSTATIC AGENTS Place the letter of the drug in the space provided by the description. Each letter is used only once.

A. Absorbable gelatin	____ Bovine origin, nonwoven web or loose fibrous form, applied dry
B. Absorbable collagen	____ Used to cauterize and neutralize
C. Microfibrillar collagen	____ Not soluble, powder or compressed pad dipped in saline, epinephrine, or thrombin
D. Oxytocin	____ Adrenal hormone, causes vasoconstriction
E. Oxidized cellulose	____ Absorbable sponges applied dry, activates coagulation
F. Phenol and Alcohol	____ Hormone produced by the pituitary, causes uterine contractions
G. Epinephrine	____ Enzyme from bovine blood, controls capillary bleeding
H. Thrombin	____ Like cotton or knitted strip, used dry, clots rapidly, not used on bone

MATCHING: ANTICOAGULANTS Place the letter of the drug in the space provided by the description. Each letter is used only once

A. Heparin	____ Depresses prothrombin, interferes with vitamin K
B. Coumarin	____ Coats platelets to prevent clumping
C. Low-molecular-weight dextran	____ Decreases clumping of platelets, inhibits vitamin K
D. Aspirin	____ Prolongs clotting time, not dissolve an existing clot

CRITICAL THINKING ACTIVITIES

Practice physical assessment skills: Can be performed head-to-toe or as review of systems (ROS)
- Cardiopulmonary
  Pulses, apical and peripheral. Observe for quality, rate, rhythm, and any difference in comparison of pulses in different areas of the body.
  Blood pressure: Should take pressure in both arms
  Lung sounds: bilateral, anterior, and posterior
- Overall physical appearance of the patient: Integument: skin color, temperature, texture, and hydration
- Review of other body systems: Neurologic, gastrointestinal, endocrine, and reproductive (if applicable: pregnancy, IUD, or oral contraceptives)
- Physical activities, level of consciousness, comfort, sensorium

SUMMARY OF CHAPTER 23

Blood loss prevention is preferred over blood loss replacement. Considering that Jehovah's Witnesses do not accept blood transfusions and most do not accept salvaged autologous blood either, isn't it more appropriate to prevent a potential problem by detecting a volume deficiency before it becomes critical? Patient assessment and blood loss estimation is crucial to prevention of volume related problems.

Other hemopoietic-related conditions are manageable to a certain extent if the patient has adequate preoperative preparation and assessment throughout the perioperative period.

CHAPTER 24 — WOUND CLOSURE MATERIALS

Wound closure has been accomplished through the ages by the use of many substances including natural fibers, animal, insect, and plant material to approximate wound edges. Wound closure is most effective if initial hemostasis has been accomplished first. Approximation of tissue should not strangulate circulation because decreased circulation causes devitalized tissue. Devitalized tissue has little or no circulation and therefore does not have the perfusion necessary for wound remodeling.

LEARNING OBJECTIVES

- Identify differences in anatomic tissue layers that are approximated or ligated by suture material.
- Identify differences in wound closure materials.

COMPETENCY-BASED KNOWLEDGE

- Understand the mechanism of tissue response to wound closure materials.
- Understand the patient-based factors that affect the choice of wound closure materials.
- Understand the concept of tissue approximation, not strangulation, in wound closure.
- List several characteristics of the ideal suture material.
- List several methods of wound closure other than suture.

COMPETENCY-BASED SKILL

- Demonstrate the preparation of suture for use in the surgical field.
- Demonstrate the correct methods of using suturing instrumentation.

STUDY QUESTIONS

1. The Halsted wound closure technique includes:
2. Define epithelialization.
3. Name the layers of abdominal closure.
4. What are some considerations in suture selection?
5. What knowledge should the scrub person have about suture?
6. What actions are appropriate when loading a needle onto a needleholder?
7. What are some of the advantages to using surgical staples?
8. What is the main purpose of bone grafting?
9. An elderly patient has had a total hip replacement and the excised femoral head is being preserved for homogenous bone graft. What procedures render it safe for use as a homologous bone graft?
10. What is the purpose of the Safe Medical Devices Act of 1990?

CRITICAL THINKING ACTIVITIES

1. Create a permanent poster display for the classroom or learning lab that has a sample of each style of needle and suture listed by type used in the surgical services department of the sponsoring clinical environment. Suggest not using needles that have been exposed to blood or body fluids for reasons of infection control. A second set of permanent posters could include alternative wound closure devices, such as wound strips and staples.
2. Practice arming and passing needleholders (left and right handed) via hand-to-hand and no touch/hands free techniques. Exercise caution not to puncture fingers with the needle. Discuss why accountability for sharps on the field should include always keeping needles attached to needleholders and only giving a new needle when the used needle is returned.
3. If available, try to suture with endoscopic trial equipment. It is important to understand the complexity of dexterity needed for endoscopic suturing.

SUMMARY OF CHAPTER 24

Consider that the patient may judge his or her surgical outcome based on visual scars. Most patients will ask questions such as "how many stitches do I have?". The patient cannot see the delicate work inside where a major organ repair took place. They only see the external wound closure. By this they may determine the quality of the entire surgical procedure.

SECTION NINE: POSTOPERATIVE CARE OF THE PATIENT AND THE ENVIRONMENT

CHAPTER 25 SURGICAL WOUNDS: FACTORS INFLUENCING HEALING AND INFECTION

Postoperative wound infection can cause complications that interfere with the outcome of the initial surgical procedure. Often, wound infections necessitate additional procedures, such as incision and drainage or debridement. Other complications may ensue, such as underlying herniation, dehiscence, or evisceration. Simple separation of the wound edges during the healing process signals potential complications. Many factors influence healing and frequently problems can be avoided just by practicing aseptic technique, providing adequate nutrition, and structurally supporting the wound site.

Aseptic technique prevents or impedes microbial invasion. Keeping microbial counts to an irreducible minimum offers a chance for optimal wound healing. Nutritional components help the body's natural healing mechanisms by providing physiologic building blocks for tissue remodeling. Proteins, vitamins, and minerals shape the composite necessary for epithelialization. Wound structural support is dependent on anatomic site of the incision or injury, closure materials, dressings and/or splints, and prosthetics and/or appliances used.

LEARNING OBJECTIVES

- Identify tissue layers specific to anatomic site of a wound.
- Identify several types of wound dressings and how they affect wound healing.

COMPETENCY-BASED KNOWLEDGE

- Understand wound healing mechanisms.
- Understand how extrinsic factors influence wound healing.
- Understand how intrinsic factors influence wound healing.

COMPETENCY-BASED SKILL

- Demonstrate aseptic technique in application of dressing material.
- Demonstrate the key points of wound assessment.

STUDY QUESTIONS

MATCHING: Each letter is used only once

A. Dead space	___ Inflammatory lesion in response to foreign body
B. Dehiscence	___ Immune response of body to tissue injury or foreign substance
C. Extravasation	___ Air separation between layers of wound
D. Granulation tissue	___ Decreased blood supply to tissue
E. Granuloma	___ Protrusion of underlying structure through one or more layers of wound
F. Ischemia	___ Collection of blood in tissue
G. Necrosis	___ Protrusion of organs through a wound to exterior of body
H. Seroma	___ Partial or total splitting open or separation of layers of wound
I. Herniation	___ Death of tissue
J. Tensile strength	___ Passage of blood, serum, or lymph into tissues
K. Hematoma	___ Collection of extravasated serum from interstitial tissue
L. Tissue reaction	___ Formation of fibrous collagen to fill gaps between edges of wound
M. Evisceration	___ Ability of tissue to resist rupture

1. Describe the direction of wound healing.
2. What is the most common cause of wound infection?
3. When are the first signs of wound infection most likely to be noticeable?
4. What are the signs of a possible wound infection?
5. Describe the resolution of a wound infection.
6. List four advantages of wound healing by first intention (primary union)?
7. List the reasons a wound is allowed to heal by secondary intention.
8. What preexisting health considerations may interfere in wound healing?
9. When is the wound assigned a classification and why?
10. List several reasons a nasogastric tube is frequently inserted at the beginning of a gastrointestinal surgical procedure.
11. List several ways a drain can enhance wound healing.
12. What are some of the functions of a dressing?
13. What are some of the causes of adhesions?
14. What is the purpose of infection control?
15. What preventative measures should be followed in reducing postoperative wound infections?

CRITICAL THINKING ACTIVITIES

Diagram the layers of tissue in several different areas of the body. For example, the abdominal layers differ from the layers associated with an extremity. Areas, such as a graft site, will have variations in layering. Identify at least four areas of the body where the layers differ in composition and list the component parts. These layers may also include implanted tissue substitutes or structural reinforcement. *Some examples include: abdomen, dorsal body surface, joints, cranium, anterior neck, limb, perineum, eye, thorax, oropharynx, or face.*

INTEGUMENTARY SYSTEM The skin is the largest organ system, 18 square feet, average weight 6 lbs (2.7kg). The heaviest organ, but not the largest in surface area. A 25¢ size piece of skin contains 1 yard of blood vessels, 4 yards of nerve fibers, 25 nerve endings, 100 sweat glands, and 3 million cells.

ANATOMY OF SKIN: LAYERS OF CONNECTIVE TISSUE AND ACCESSORY ORGANS

Epidermis - cutaneous outer layer; squamous /stratified epithelium 4 to 5 layers, no organs, nerve endings, or vessels.
1. Surface is keratin
2. Contains melanin

Dermis - middle layer; key layer for proper wound repair, above the adipose, easily identified and provides an anchoring site for superficial and deep sutures. Any debridement must go to this subcuticular layer.
1. Blood vessels
2. Nerve endings
3. Hair follicles
4. Glands

Adipose - subcuticular layer above the fascia, protects from heat loss, padding against trauma. Devitalized tissue in this layer leads to infection and ischemia easily.
1. Blood vessels
2. Glands
3. Hair follicles

Fascia - superficial and deep fibrous layers overlie muscle
1. Injection of local anesthetic should extend between the dermis and superficial fascia.
2. Deep fascia supports the superficial layers and encases the muscles. Any injury to this layer should be sutured to ensure the integrity of the underlying layers.

Appendages to the integument
1. Hair follicles are ingrowths of epidermis, hair and nails are hard keratin, modified epidermis.
2. Arrector pili - smooth muscle attached to follicle
3. Glands
   a. Sebaceous oil glands - single duct with 4-5 sacculated organs, greatest in number on face, scalp, and natural body openings. Produces lubricant. Open into hair follicle. Largest glands are on the eyelids.
      1. holocrine glands - release whole cells full of sebum
   b. Sudoriferous sweat glands - waste excretion aqueous and gaseous material, cooling by evaporation
      1. eccrine - open directly to skin surfaces, general body surface area, secrete in response to physical activity
      2. apocrine - open into hair follicle, mostly genital and axillary, secrete in response to stress or excitation
4. Nails - ungues (plural), consist of a root, body, and free edge. Arises from the matrix (nailbed) and overlies the corium of the digit tip. Grows to the tip of the digit in a series of grooves.

PHYSIOLOGY OF THE INTEGUMENT
1. Protection - barrier, waterproof cover, pigment protects from ultraviolet light

2. Regulates body temperature as a constant internal environment
3. Regenerates
4. Absorbs some good things, such as lanolins and medications and bad things, such as toxins
5. Tactile sense is a communication device
6. General health indicator through appearance and texture
7. Excretion of metabolic waste
8. Secretion ports
9. Produces some vitamin D in the presence of sunlight
10. Contributes to sense of self-esteem and well-being; can convey beauty and ugliness

INFLAMMATION (Not to be confused with infection) This process is a natural body defense and is beneficial in the event of injury by creating a natural bandage, splint, or immobilizer. Prepares the body for repair and restoration. Happens only in living tissue with intact circulation, action is to inactivate an offending agent. Inflammation can be local or systemic. Local reactions may signify a wound infection. Systemic reactions may signal a septic, potentially serious condition.

CARDINAL SIGNS OF INFLAMMATION

Local reactions	Systemic reactions
Red	Flushed
Hot	Fever
Swollen	Edema, generalized
Pain	Somatic aches
Altered function	Dizziness; weakness

INFLUENCES ON WOUND HEALING: ASSESSMENT OF RISK FACTORS
Most wounds will progress to natural healing unless infected, poor closure, devitalization, or interrupted by other outside influences.
1. Age, general health, mobility, length of procedure
   - Dermal-epidermal planes flatten causing decreased vascularity of aging tissue; tensile strength decreases causing the surface to tear and injure easily; low resistance to suture tension; should reinforce wounds with wound closure strips in elderly
2. Nutritional status
   - Alcoholism interferes with nutrition and impacts wound healing
   - Obesity usually indicates poor nutrition and influences wound healing
3. Foreign body, infection, dead space
4. Circulatory status, respiratory status, oxygenation, chronic hypoxia, anemia, peripheral vascular disease
5. Endocrine and immunological status, diabetes, hereditary factors
6. Radiation, disease process, surgical technique (laser, electrosurgery); devitalized tissue
7. Type of closure used (suture, staples, tape strips), poor wound prep, tension on wound, type of suture, local anesthetics with vasoconstrictors added; tissue handling
8. The amount of tissue lost or removed, innervation (true depth and lateral extent)
9. Medications - Anticoagulants, anti-inflammatory, chemo, colchicine, corticosteroids
10. Uremia

11. Anatomic site: head and neck have less infections than extremities; wounds across joints have more contractures
12. How the wound was actually created; was it a controlled surgical incision or a traumatic tear?
13. Degree of contamination
14. Drains used

COMPLICATIONS THAT AFFECT WOUND HEALING

Hemorrhage / hematoma can impair or interrupt circulation and provide a basis for infection

Infection - abscess in solid tissue, can tunnel; microorganism present, could be anaerobic, aerobic or facultative organism; greater incidence in over 50 y/o who has diabetes, malnourished, and steroids

Disruptions of wound that would delay healing
- Disruption - shortly after surgery the wound loses integrity, coughing, etc
- Dehiscence - wound edges open or separate unexpectedly 5-8 days postoperatively, may signify an infection, culture any exudate
- Evisceration - wound edges open unexpectedly, contents such as internal organs extrude through the opening
- Fistula - abnormal tunnel or passage between two organs
- Sinus tract - abnormal tunnel or passage to outside of body
- Fissure - abnormal tear or split in tissue at an orifice
- Incisional hernia - opening of sub-layers of a previous surgical site; the skin usually remains closed, but a bulge is present and palpable

Scar / cicatrix: Influenced by proximity to lines of dynamic tension
- Adhesions - undesired filmy bands of scar tissue that bind organs together
- Keloid - over sized, hypertrophied scar tissue; mostly in dark skinned people
- Hypertrophied scar - over areas of stress, like joints
- Contracture - disuse and scar tissue causes shortening of muscles, nerves, ligaments, and tendons; affected part assumes a retained position of non function
- Neuroma - nerve endings encased in scar tissue, palpable mass
- Granuloma - foreign object / body (FB) walled off, body unable to absorb the FB particle

Ulcer - chronic irritation
- Mechanical - friction causes tissue breakdown
- Chemical - gastric acids, enzymes, environmental waste
- Stasis ulcer - occluded venous circulation causes tissue aseptic necrosis
- Ischemic ulcer - occluded arterial circulation causes tissue breakdown

ASSESSING THE WOUND: OBSERVATIONS
- Patient and family/significant other's awareness of wound healing influences and risk factors
- Potential for microbial contamination
- Color, swelling, pain, temperature, drainage (amount, color, consistency, and odor), any unexpected observational difference, and any complaint by the patient

CONSIDERATIONS
- Location and size of the wound

- Who will be caring for the wound, socioeconomics, education
- The potential for infection
- The manner of healing and dressing employed
- Preferences of the surgeon
- Medications and nutritional influences
- Affect and participation of the patient in self-care

SUMMARY OF CHAPTER 25

The wound is a key link to the success of the surgical procedure. Structurally, the surgical wound was the access point to the primary working area of the OR team. Psychologically to the patient, the visible portions of the wound are constant reminders of the experience. Patients may measure a large part of the success of the procedure on the appearance of the incision. Closure is important as described in Chapter 24, but complications of the wound, such as infection or disruption can have both psychologic and physiologic impact. Prevention of problems offers the best opportunity to meet expected outcomes without untoward effects.

CHAPTER 26   POSTOPERATIVE PATIENT CARE

The postoperative period of care for a patient who has received general anesthesia is much like caring for an intensive care patient. When the procedure is complete, and anesthesia has been reversed, the patient is vulnerable to serious and complex physiologically mediated complications. Caregivers need to be attentive to the patient and the anesthesia provider and consider that this period of time may be extremely critical as the patient transcends the intraoperative phase of care into the postoperative period. As discussed in previous chapters, the setup should remain sterile until the patient has been taken to the postanesthesia unit (PACU). Often in an effort to move the surgical schedule forward, the OR team, particularly the circulator, finds it necessary to prepare for subsequent patients before the current patient has left the room. This practice may take significant attention away from a potentially critical situation and place the patient in jeopardy.

Postoperative patient care phases as defined by ASPAN are described in Chapter 26 of the main text, but can be further defined as five more distinct phases. These phases are dependent on the complexity of the anesthetic, the surgical procedure, and the overall condition of the patient. As the critical nature of the patient's condition lessens, the patient's level of care decreases. Throughout each of these five phases of care, the attainment of expected outcomes is measured and the plan of care modified according to the patient's ongoing assessment. The amount of time in each phase will vary according to institutional protocol and patient condition. The times listed are examples of relative time frames.

1. *Immediate postoperative phase*: The period of time when maintenance of anesthesia is concluded and reversal begins. The dressing is applied, the patient is placed on a transport stretcher, and the patient is taken out of the OR. (20-30 minutes)
2. *Transitory postoperative phase*: The period of time during which the patient has exited the OR, is being transported to the postanesthesia care area, and postoperative report is exchanged between caregivers. Should be accompanied by anesthesia provider and perioperative nurse. Physiologic condition is monitored throughout the exchange of information. (15-20 minutes)
3. *Progressive postoperative phase*: The period of time during which the patient becomes increasingly stable, regains use of natural protective reflexes, and is taken from the postanesthesia care area to the patient care division for further care or discharge from the facility. (30 minutes to several hours)
4. *Postoperative stabilization phase*: The period of time during which the patient remains in the care of caregivers in a patient care division. (several hours or several days)
5. *Remote postoperative phase*: The period of time during which the patient is capable of release from the facility and able to perform self-care activities or care can be transferred to a less acute environment. Some facilities offer follow-up telephone calls to patients in their homes. Postoperative care instructions may be given in written form to patient and/or other caregiver. (several hours or several weeks)

LEARNING OBJECTIVES

- Identify potential complications that can take place in the postoperative period.
- List the salient facts that should be included in the postoperative report to the PACU nurse.
- List several considerations for giving a postoperative report to the PACU nurse about various patient populations, such as pediatric, geriatric, or other special needs patient.

COMPETENCY-BASED KNOWLEDGE

- Understand each caregiver's role in the care of the postoperative patient.
- Understand the responsibility of the OR team in the care of a patient who has died in the OR.
- Understand the importance of handling protocols for forensic evidence.

COMPETENCY-BASED SKILL

- Demonstrate verbal skill in delivering postoperative report to the PACU nurse.
- Demonstrate the procedure for initial admission assessment in PACU.

STUDY QUESTIONS

1. What determines the patient's length of stay in the postanesthesia care unit?
2. Who is responsible for discharging patients from PACU?
3. When evaluating expected outcomes postoperatively, what considerations should the perioperative nurse include?
4. List the complications arising from the administration of anesthesia.
5. List the standard monitoring equipment needed at each bedside in PACU.
6. Care of the postoperative surgical patient, who is 7 months pregnant, should include assessment and monitoring of:
7. List the important components of the postoperative report to the PACU nurse.
8. PACU nurses should be certified in Basic Life Support, Cardiopulmonary Resuscitation, and Advance Cardiac Life Support. TRUE / FALSE
9. What determines the postmortem care of a patient who expires in the operating room?
10. What is considered forensic evidence?
11. How should forensic evidence be stored for release to the Coroner's office?
12. What responsibilities does the circulator have in giving after-death care in the OR?

CRITICAL THINKING ACTIVITIES

Outline the main components of postoperative care for different patient populations. Take into consideration age, general health status, safety issues, and other patient-specific characteristics. Comparisons may be made to Chapters 7, 8, 42, 43, 44, and 45 of the main text and this resource manual for information and contrasts between specific patient populations.
- Pediatric patient
- Geriatric patient

- Adolescent patient
- Terminal patient
- Pregnant, nonobstetric surgical patient

SUMMARY OF CHAPTER 26

The perioperative experience begins with the preoperative assessment of the patient and the development of the plan of care by the perioperative nurse. The full circle of events culminates with the postoperative phase and the transition to a state of wellness or improvement supported by the purpose of the surgical procedure. The processes involved with the flow of perioperative events should benefit and not harm the patient. This is the focus of attainment of expected outcomes. All outcomes are not fully measurable until the patient has been released from care. Untoward events may still affect the patient after release from the OR. For some patients, this is the most critical turning point of the perioperative care cycle.

Postoperative observation of the patient significantly improves the attainment of expected outcomes. The plan of care is evaluated and many nursing diagnoses are resolved. Prevention of complications, patient education, and health maintenance are features of the postoperative phase of care.

CHAPTER 27   POSTOPERATIVE CARE OF THE PHYSICAL ENVIRONMENT

Environmental contamination can be a source of infection to both caregivers and patients. Sources of environmental contamination may include people, supplies, equipment, insects, packaging materials, and anything that is not specifically intrinsic to the actual patient receiving care. Any surface, living or inanimate, can serve as a vector or carrier for a harmful substance. Contaminants include microorganisms, chemicals, foreign particulate matter, and other materials that can interfere with the health and safety of the patient and team. Aseptic technique targets microorganisms, but as a side benefit, maintaining a clean, safe environment also eliminates or decreases the effects of other potentially injurious materials. Chemicals and other harmful substances listed in the material safety data sheets (MSDS) sheets are treated accordingly as discussed in Chapter 10.

LEARNING OBJECTIVES

- Identify areas of personnel, equipment, and room that are considered contaminated during and after the procedure.
- Identify potential sources of wound contamination other than microorganisms.

COMPETENCY-BASED KNOWLEDGE

- Understand the difference between care of the environment before, during, and after a surgical procedure.

COMPETENCY-BASED SKILL

- Demonstrate the procedures for environmental care before a surgical procedure, such as first case of the day and between case cleanup.
- Demonstrate the procedure for environmental care during a surgical procedure.
- Demonstrate the procedure for environmental care after a surgical procedure.
- Demonstrate the procedure for terminal room care.

STUDY QUESTIONS

1. Every patient is considered a potential contaminant. TRUE /FALSE
2. Before discarding any drapes, what should the scrub nurse check for?
3. At what point should the scrub person break down the sterile field?
4. How should blades be removed from the knife handles? Where should they be discarded?
5. Describe the procedure for taking care of the instruments after the surgical procedure.
6. List the personnel, equipment, and areas that are considered contaminated during and after the surgical procedure.
7. Describe the method used to remove contaminated gloves.

8. When is terminal cleaning of the OR performed?

CRITICAL THINKING ACTIVITIES

Create a chart that lists potential contaminants and their effects on the patient and caregivers. Substances may include microorganisms, chemicals, vapors, body substances, particulates, and other vectors.

SUMMARY OF CHAPTER 27

Environmental contamination is not limited to microorganisms. Cleaning procedures throughout the work day should be thorough enough to afford protection from other potentially harmful substances that could interfere with the well-being of the patient and OR team.

SECTION TEN: SURGICAL SPECIALTIES

The following surgical specialties in Chapters 28 through 40 include learning objectives and critical thinking exercises specific to each body system and the organs involved. Competency based knowledge and skill is applied directly to technique-oriented practice and is not isolated in each surgical service to avoid redundancy of material. References to previous technique-oriented chapters in the main text and the resource manual are included as needed for emphasis.

CHAPTER 28   DIAGNOSTIC PROCEDURES

LEARNING OBJECTIVES

- Identify several diagnostic procedures that are performed before surgical intervention.
- Identify several noninvasive radiologic diagnostic procedures performed before surgical intervention.
- Identify several invasive diagnostic procedures performed before surgical intervention.
- List several pre- and intra- radiologic procedural patient care considerations.
- Identify several varieties of radiopaque contrast media used for diagnostic procedures.
- List the signs and symptoms of adverse reaction to radiopaque contrast media.
- Describe the care of a patient who is having an adverse reaction to radiopaque contrast media.
- Demonstrate the precautions taken for patient and personnel safety during a radiologic procedure.

STUDY QUESTIONS

1. What are the four main classifications of diagnostic procedures?
2. List eight diagnostic modalities used for diagnosing conditions in perioperative patients.
3. List several types of pathologic testing used to establish a diagnosis.
4. List several noninvasive imaging studies.
5. List the conditions in which conventional x-ray is useful in diagnosing.
6. List several invasive diagnostic studies.
7. What are the signs and symptoms of an adverse reaction to contrast media?
8. What are the key factors in minimizing radiation exposure for patient and OR team?
9. List several applications of intraoperative ultrasound.
10. List several therapeutic functions of intraoperative endoscopy.

Identify whether the diagnostic procedure is invasive or noninvasive.

I = INVASIVE N = NONINVASIVE	
___ Biopsy	___ Culture
___ Chest x-ray	___ Mammogram
___ Fluoroscopy	___ Arthrogram
___ Cardiac catheterization	___ Doppler
___ Endoscopy	___ PET scan
___ Ultrasound	___ Pulse oximetry
___ Sensory evoked potential	___ CT scan with contrast
___ Retrograde pyelogram	___ Cholangiogram

CRITICAL THINKING ACTIVITIES

Create a list of several pathologic conditions for each body system in the form of provisional or preliminary diagnoses. Identify the signs and symptoms that would possibly be observed with each diagnoses. List the diagnostic tests, both invasive and/or noninvasive, that may be performed to finalize the patient's diagnosis. This exercise may extend into each of the surgical specialty chapters as a continued exercise. Suggestions include:

1. Formulating the material in chart form with a column for each aspect of the condition and diagnostics. The information can flow into therapeutics and/or surgical intervention, followed by prognostics.
2. Maintaining a separate notebook with a divider for each surgical specialty with the above described format.
3. Starting a journal club within the learning group. Each learner is assigned a surgical specialty to collect articles and references of current material for presentation and distribution within the learning group. Refer also to Chapter 1 of this resource manual for information about performing a computer search for the collection of references and journal articles. Consult with the librarian of the clinical site for assistance in performing a computer search through Medline (National Library of Medicine, Bethesda, Maryland). Most libraries have access to this collection of databases.

CHAPTER 29   GENERAL SURGERY

LEARNING OBJECTIVES

- Identify the pertinent anatomy of abdominal organs within the peritoneal cavity.
- Identify six types of abdominal incisions used in general surgery.
- Describe preoperative preparation of a patient for gastrointestinal surgery.
- Identify the procedures performed for the four stages of breast cancer.
- List several complications that could occur in abdominal surgery.
- Demonstrate patient positioning for open abdominal surgery.
- Demonstrate patient positioning for an abdominal laparoscopic procedure.
- List the technical principles for gastrointestinal anastomoses.

STUDY QUESTIONS

1. Breast biopsy for cytologic testing may be performed by:
2. Removal of the entire breast, resection of all axillary lymph nodes, and possibly the pectoralis minor muscle is called:
3. Removal of the entire breast tumor mass with surrounding nondiseased tissue is called:
4. Which incision is primarily used for exposure of the superior aspect of the stomach and inferior aspect of the esophagus?
5. What is an open incision for an appendectomy made just below the umbilicus and 4cm medial from the anterior iliac spine?
6. List three common areas of the intestines for creation of stomas
7. Name the incision most commonly used for an inguinal hernia.
8. What are the organ functions that form and secrete bile, transforms glucose into glycogen, and helps to regulate blood clotting?
9. List several open surgical procedures that are also performed as minimally invasive laparoscopic procedures.
10. Chronic gastric, pyloric, and duodenal ulcers can benefit from the interruption of the vagus nerve. This procedure is called:

MATCHING: Match column A with column B. Each letter is used only once.

Procedure	Organ
A. Hepatectomy	___ Colon
B. Splenectomy	___ Gall bladder
C. Appendectomy	___ Hemorrhoids
D. Mastectomy	___ Liver
E. Herniorrhaphy	___ Appendix
F. Gastrectomy	___ Breast
G. Cholecystectomy	___ Spleen
H. Colectomy	___ Supporting musculature
I. Hemorrhoidectomy	___ Stomach

CRITICAL THINKING ACTIVITIES

Identify the advantages and disadvantages of general laparoscopic procedures to open procedures. For example, compare an open cholecystectomy with a laparoscopic cholecystectomy. For open procedures and minimally invasive approaches, list preoperative teaching and preparation of the patient, intraoperative considerations, and postoperative follow-up. Include consideration of financial aspects, such as return to work or continued care.

CHAPTER 30   GYNECOLOGY AND OBSTETRICS

LEARNING OBJECTIVES

- Identify the anatomy of the female urinary system.
- Identify the anatomy of the female reproductive system.
- Understand the physiology of the female reproductive system.
- Identify several common diagnostic procedures used in gynecologic practice.
- List the rationale for performing a vaginal hysterectomy versus an abdominal hysterectomy.
- List the equipment necessary in the OR when performing a cesarean section.
- Understand the differences in procedures performed to correct urinary stress incontinence. in the female patient
- Demonstrate the positioning techniques that should be used when placing a patient in the lithotomy position for a gynecologic procedure.
- Demonstrate the table setup with instrumentation for a dilatation and curettage procedure.

STUDY QUESTIONS

1. Which diagnostic techniques involves staining cervical squamous epithelium with iodine-based Lugol's solution?
2. Cancer of the cervix is diagnosed most often in association with:
3. Rubin's test (uterotubal insufflation), used to test patency of the fallopian tubes, should follow uterine curettage. TRUE / FALSE
4. Pelvic endoscopy is not a sterile procedure. TRUE / FALSE
5. What may cause postoperative pain following use of pneumoperitoneum for laparoscopy?
6. List several procedures used to treat severe dysplasia and/or carcinoma of the cervix in situ.
7. Removal of the fallopian tubes is called:
8. Describe pelvic exenteration.
9. Intraperitoneal adhesions following pelvic surgery may cause:
10. Describe cerclage by the Shirodkar procedure.
11. Which uterine incision used for cesarean section causes less intraoperative blood loss and chance of rupture with subsequent pregnancies?
12. What signs and symptoms characterize an ectopic pregnancy?

MATCHING: Each letter is used only once.

Condition	Definition
A. Ectopic pregnancy	____ Herniated bladder into vagina
B. Endometriosis	____ Removal of ovary
C. Salpingitis	____ Benign mass of uterus
D. Corpus luteal cyst	____ Removal of uterus
E. Endometrioma	____ Aberrant endometrial tissue
F. Fibroid uterus	____ Inflammation of fallopian tube
G. Cystocele	____ Gestation outside of uterus
H. Oophorectomy	____ Follicular cyst of ovary
I. Hysterectomy	____ Mass of endometrial tissue

CRITICAL THINKING ACTIVITIES

Create a case study based on an actual or simulated obstetric patient who experiences complications necessitating a cesarean section for delivery. The case study should include information about the entire course of the gestation, preoperative, intraoperative and postoperative considerations for the mother and her fetus, and expected outcomes of perinatal care.

CHAPTER 31 UROLOGIC SURGERY

LEARNING OBJECTIVES

- Identify the pertinent anatomy of the male urinary system.
- Identify the pertinent anatomy of the male reproductive system.
- Compare the differences of male and female urinary system anatomy.
- Compare the various endoscopes used for urologic procedures.
- Understand the differences between hemodialysis and peritoneal dialysis.
- Describe the procedures performed to treat a patient with urolithiasis.
- Describe the procedures performed to correct urinary incontinence.
- Describe the procedures performed for treatment of prostatic cancer.
- Describe the procedures performed for urinary diversion.

STUDY QUESTIONS

1. What causes renal damage?
2. Which structure is the essential working unit of the kidney?
3. The size of urologic endoscopes are measured in which scale?
4. Cystoscopy includes examination of what anatomic areas?
5. Describe the location of the prostate gland.
6. Which are the main functions of renal dialysis?
7. Surgical approaches to access the kidney include which incisions?
8. Describe surgical excision of the prostate and the postoperative implications for the patient.
9. Male impotence can be surgically treated by which procedures?
10. Anastomosis of the vas deferens is performed for what reason?

MATCHING: Each letter is used only once.

Condition	Definition
A. Nephrolithiasis	____ Dilation of spermatic veins
B. Pyelitis	____ Removal of testis
C. Prostatic hypertrophy	____ Accumulated fluid in scrotum
D. Epididymitis	____ Anastomosis of vas deferens
E. Varicocele	____ Calculi in kidney
F. Cystitis	____ Inflammation of kidney pelvis
G. Orchiectomy	____ Enlarged prostate
H. Hydrocele	____ Inflamed urinary bladder
I. Vasovasostomy	____ Inflammation of seminal passage

CRITICAL THINKING ACTIVITIES

Create a case study outlining the perioperative course of an actual or simulated patient who has prostatic cancer and is scheduled to have a radical prostatectomy. Include consideration for diagnostic procedures, perioperative care, and psychosocial implications.

CHAPTER 32   ORTHOPAEDIC SURGERY

LEARNING OBJECTIVES

- Identify the pertinent anatomy of the musculoskeletal system.
- Identify several different types of fractures and their stabilization for the healing process.
- Understand the differences between internal and external fixation procedures.
- Identify the main components of a prosthetic hip joint.
- Demonstrate how to mix cement for a prosthetic hip joint.
- Demonstrate how to assemble power equipment.
- Understand the safe use and handling of casting material.

STUDY QUESTIONS

1. List the functions of the musculoskeletal system.
2. List several causes of osteomyelitis.
3. List the effects of osteomyelitis on bone healing.
4. Which lasers are used for arthroscopic procedures?
5. What substance is used to provide hemostasis in bone?
6. Laminar airflow is used to create an ultra-clean environment for orthopaedic surgery? TRUE / FALSE
7. List several intraoperative protective recommendations of the American Academy of Orthopaedic Surgeons.
8. How can spinal stabilization may be accomplished?
9. Outline the stages of osteogenesis (bone formation and healing).
10. Describe the Ilizarov technique for salvaging infected and non-union fractures.
11. List several types of tissue that may be treated through the arthroscope.

MATCHING: Each letter is used only once.

Condition	Definition
A. Osteomyelitis	___ Lateral deviation of great toe
B. Malunion	___ Supportive dressing material
C. Synovitis	___ Separation of joint
D. Open fracture	___ Surgical fusion of joint
E. Osteogenesis	___ Bone fails to heal correctly
F. Cast	___ Infection of bone
G. Arthrodesis	___ Broken bone protrudes through skin
H. Dislocation	___ New bone growth
I. Hallux valgus	___ Inflammation of joint capsule

CRITICAL THINKING ACTIVITIES

Create a case study of a patient having a total joint arthroplasty procedure. Include pre-, intra-, and postoperative considerations for the patient's care. Patient and significant others' instruction and discharge planning should be included. Identify expected outcomes.

CHAPTER 33 — OPHTHALMIC SURGERY

LEARNING OBJECTIVES

- Identify the pertinent anatomy of the eye and surrounding structures.
- List the procedures performed on the eye for the treatment of glaucoma.
- Identify the differences between extracapsular and intracapsular extraction of the lens.
- List the advantages and disadvantages of intraocular lens implantation.
- List the various traumas and their treatments that could occur to the eye.
- Understand the actions of mydriatic and miotic drugs.
- Understand the different methods of anesthetizing the eye using local anesthesia.
- Demonstrate the preoperative preparation of an ophthalmic surgery patient.

STUDY QUESTIONS

1. What is the mucous membrane that lines the inner side of the eyelids and the exposed surface of the sclera, except the cornea?
2. What is the visual component consisting of clear transparent gelatinous protein encased in a capsule supported by suspensory ligaments?
3. List the three main causes of blindness.
4. Name the benign, oil-secreting cyst of the eyelid.
5. Drooping of the eyelid is called:
6. Dacryocystectomy involves removal of what structure?
7. Removal of the entire eyeball is called:
8. Which term best describes a full-thickness corneal transplant?
9. Describe the characteristics of glaucoma.
10. Describe the characteristics of a cataract.
11. Fluorescein angiography is used to visualize which structure?
12. Describe the characteristics of retinal detachment.
13. Describe the functional components of vision.

MATCHING: Each letter is used only once.

Condition	Definition
A. Ptosis	___ Excise a small section of the iris
B. Pterygium	___ Tearing away
C. Keratotomy	___ Droop
D. Chalazion	___ Cloudy lens
E. Keratoplasty	___ Pneumopexy of retina
F. Iridectomy	___ Mydriasis
G. Cataract	___ Repair of cornea
H. Gas tamponade	___ Cyst of Meibomian gland
I. Vitrectomy	___ Incisions into cornea
J. Avulsion	___ Tissue overgrowth onto cornea
K. Dilation of pupil	___ Removal of vitreous

CRITICAL THINKING ACTIVITIES

Create a case study based on a corneal transplant patient. Include perioperative consideration for accommodation of decreased vision and the care needed by the patient after surgery.

CHAPTER 34   PLASTIC AND RECONSTRUCTIVE SURGERY

LEARNING OBJECTIVES

- Identify the pertinent anatomic structures of the integumentary system.
- Describe four classifications of burns in relation to the anatomic layers of the skin.
- Identify four main reasons for plastic surgery.
- Identify several types of grafting techniques.
- Understand the importance of psychologic support for the patient undergoing plastic surgery.
- Understand the significance of vascularization of grafted tissue.
- Explain the importance of fluid replacement in a burn patient.
- Demonstrate the prevention and care of pressure ulcers.

STUDY QUESTIONS

1. List four reasons to perform plastic surgery.
2. New skin is generated by which layer of the integument?
3. Pedicle flaps consist of which tissue layers and structures?
4. What adjustable instrument is used to excise free skin grafts?
5. Full-thickness skin grafts consist of which tissue layers?
6. Split-thickness grafts consist of which tissue layers?
7. A split-thickness skin graft can be adapted for a larger surface area by what process?
8. Myocutaneous flaps include the components of pedicle flaps in addition to which other structures?
9. What process increases tissue for coverage of a large surface area?
10. Following a modified or radical mastectomy list several considerations for successful breast reconstruction.
11. Outline several psychologic considerations of plastic surgery.

MATCHING: Each letter is used only once.

Condition	Definition
A. Rhytidectomy	___ Aspiration of adipose tissue
B. Rhinoplasty	___ Layered excision of skin cancer
C. Blepharoplasty	___ Securing edges of rectus muscle
D. Otoplasty	___ Scar revision
E. Liposuction	___ Nose reshaping
F. Mastopexy	___ Skin resurfacing
G. Panniculectomy	___ Ear reconstruction
H. Plication	___ Removal of excess eyelid skin
I. Z-plasty	___ Removal of loose facial skin
J. Moh's micrograph	___ Elevation of sagging breast tissue
K. Dermabrasion	___ Removal of excess abdominal skin

CRITICAL THINKING ACTIVITIES

Create a case study based on a patient who was born with multiple congenital deformities and plans to undergo multiple surgical procedures in more than one surgical discipline. Outline each procedure complete with expected outcomes. Identify the psychologic implications of pre-, intra-, and postoperative phase of care. Simulate an evaluation of the plan of care.

CHAPTER 35   OTORHINOLARYNGOLOGY: ENT SURGERY

LEARNING OBJECTIVES

- Identify the pertinent anatomy of the ear.
- Identify the pertinent anatomy of the nasopharynx.
- Understand the physiology of hearing and the causes of hearing loss.
- Understand the risk factors involved in throat surgery.

STUDY QUESTIONS

1. Name the three main anatomic areas of the ear.
2. What is hearing loss most often attributed to?
3. Surgically correctable conductive hearing loss is caused by a defect in one of which two anatomic areas?
4. A bone conduction implant is a small magnetic disc which is implanted in:
5. Name the surgical procedure performed to repair defects in the eardrum is.
6. What is the removal of damaged or infected mastoid air cells called?
7. List the functions of the nose.
8. Epistaxis usually involves what structure:
9. Obstructive sleep apnea may eventually cause which life-threatening complications if untreated?
10. Which lasers are frequently used in the oropharynx?

MATCHING: Each letter is used only once.

Condition	Definition
A. Oropharynx obstruction	___ Benign tumor of 8th cranial nerve
B. Mastoiditis	___ Ossification of middle ear bones
C. Osteoma	___ Inflammation of middle ear
D. Otitis media	___ Nosebleed
E. Sensorineural deficit	___ Inflamed air cells
F. Acoustic neuroma	___ Bone tumor
G. Epistaxis	___ Enlarged uvula and soft palate
H. Otosclerosis	___ Endolymphatic excess

CRITICAL THINKING ACTIVITIES

Create a case study based on a patient who has had a serious hearing loss from a young age. Include consideration of speech patterns, safety issues, and adjustment to temporary versus permanent hearing augmentation. Determine if the patient has met expected outcomes and evaluate the plan of care.

CHAPTER 36 — HEAD AND NECK SURGERY

LEARNING OBJECTIVES

- Identify the pertinent anatomic structures of the face and neck.
- Identify the components and function of a tracheostomy tube.
- Identify several indications for performing a laryngoscopy.
- Discuss the psychosocial effects of head and neck surgery.
- Understand the psychosocial implications of a radical neck procedure for laryngeal cancer.
- Demonstrate the precautions that must be taken when performing laser microlaryngoscopy.

STUDY QUESTIONS

1. What are the risks of parotid gland surgery?
2. List two positive indications that the patient is psychosocially adapting to facial surgery.
3. List the diagnostic tools used to determine the extent of craniofacial deformity.
4. Facial fractures involve which facial bones?
5. From which area is autograft frequently taken for mandibular reconstruction?
6. Describe the orthognathic bite disorders of one or both jaws that displace the alignment of the outside of normal relationship with the cranial bones.
7. What is the removal of the tongue called?
8. List several indications for laryngoscopy.
9. List several patient care issues surrounding tracheotomy.
10. List the postoperative risks of thyroidectomy.

MATCHING: Each letter is used only once.

Condition	Definition
A. Hypertelorism	___ Tongue inflammation
B. Malar fracture	___ Inflamed closure of vocal cords
C. Articular joint dysfunction	___ Temporomandibular syndrome
D. Malocclusion	___ Jaw misalignment
E. Parotiditis	___ Inflamed salivary gland
F. Glossitis	___ Wide space between orbits
G. Epiglottitis	___ Broken zygoma

CRITICAL THINKING ACTIVITIES

Create a perioperative case study about a geriatric patient who is having a total thyroidectomy. Identify the expected outcomes and evaluate the simulated plan of care. Chapter 43 discusses perioperative considerations for the geriatric patient.

CHAPTER 37 — NEUROSURGERY

LEARNING OBJECTIVES

- Identify the pertinent anatomy of the brain and the spinal cord.
- Understand the significance of specific neurologic monitoring procedures.
- Understand the risks involved in neurosurgery.

STUDY QUESTIONS

1. Why are scalp clips used during a craniotomy?
2. List several measures performed during craniotomy to lower blood pressure, decrease cerebral blood flow and venous pressure, decrease brain volume, and prevent increased intracranial pressure.
3. List the postoperative complications of a craniotomy.
4. List the advantages of the prone position on a supportive frame to hyperextend the spine.
5. What is the division of the anterior motor roots of spinal nerves to control the involuntary muscle contractions associated with spastic paralysis called?
6. List two methods for relieving intractable pain.
7. Hypophysectomy is the removal of which structure?
8. List several types of physiologic monitoring performed during cranial procedures.
9. List three types of evoked potential monitoring used during neurologic procedures.
10. List several uses of stereotaxis as applied to neurosurgery.

MATCHING: Each letter is used only once.

Condition	Definition
A. Subdural hematoma	___ Electrical impulse-induced seizure
B. Cerebral edema	___ Pain not relieved by conventional treatment
C. Epilepsy	___ Increased fluid in ventricles of brain
D. Intractable pain	___ Abnormal vascular communication
E. Hydrocephalus	___ Bleeding between the dura and arachnoid
F. Arteriovenous malformation	___ Brain swelling

CRITICAL THINKING ACTIVITIES

Create a case study about a female patient who is having a craniotomy for a cerebral lesion. Describe the perioperative implications including the diagnostics used to detect the tumor, the psychosocial aspects of self-image, and potential hazards pre-, intra-, and postoperatively. Identify the expected outcomes and evaluate the simulated plan of care.

CHAPTER 38 — THORACIC SURGERY

LEARNING OBJECTIVES

- Identify the pertinent anatomy of the thoracic cavity.
- List the potential complications of thoracic surgery.
- Demonstrate setup and maintenance of water-seal chest drainage system.

STUDY QUESTIONS

1. The thoracic cavity contains what areas and anatomic structures?
2. A puncture of the right pleural cavity can cause the lung on the left side to collapse by what process?
3. Describe the endoscopic procedure that provides direct visualization of intrathoracic lymph nodes?
4. What are the key points to remember when setting up a thoracic water-seal chest tube drainage system?
5. Describe the functions of a water-seal chest drainage system using two chest tubes.
6. List the factors that influence the choice of incisions for thoracic surgery.
7. The primary reason for most lung resections is the presence of neoplasms. TRUE / FALSE
8. What is the physiology of a sucking chest wound?
9. Thymectomy is performed to relieve the symptoms of what disease?
10. What are some of the potential complications of thoracic surgery?

MATCHING: Each letter is used only once.

Condition	Definition
A. Hemothorax	___ Funnel chest
B. Pectus carinatum	___ Diaphragmatic bulging
C. Mediastinal shift	___ Fibrous thickening of visceral pleural membrane
D. Thoracic outlet syndrome	___ Bloody drainage in thorax
E. Hiatal hernia	___ Increased intrathoracic atmospheric pressure
F. Pectus excavatum	___ Vessel and nerve impingement at 1st rib
G. Empyema	___ Lateral movement of thoracic organs
H. Pneumothorax	___ Pigeon chest

CRITICAL THINKING ACTIVITIES

Create a case study about a patient who has had a lung resection for mixed cell carcinoma. Include preoperative diagnostics, intraoperative positioning and monitoring, and postoperative care. Describe the surgical procedure and expected outcomes. Evaluate the simulated plan of care.

CHAPTER 39   CARDIAC SURGERY

LEARNING OBJECTIVES

- Identify the pertinent anatomy of the heart and great vessels
- List the various types of grafts used for coronary artery bypass grafting
- Describe the function of a cardiac pacemaker

STUDY QUESTIONS

1. Describe the anatomy of the heart and major blood vessels supplying the heart muscle.
2. List several ways to deliberately arrest the heart.
3. What pathologic conditions cause thromboembolism associated with cardiac valvular disease.
4. Which autologous artery has the best long term patency rate?
5. Describe the direction of blood flow through saphenous vein grafts.
6. Trace the flow of blood through the heart.
7. Describe the function of the cardiac conduction system.
8. What should a circulator know about a patient that has a pacemaker scheduled for a surgical procedure using local anesthesia?
9. Describe cardiac tamponade.
10. Cardiopulmonary bypass is a temporary substitute for the patient's heart and lungs. TRUE / FALSE

MATCHING: Each letter is used only once.

Procedure	Definition
A. Endarterectomy	___ Repair dilation of the ventricular wall
B. Laser angioplasty	___ Resuscitative oxygenation in cardiopulmonary failure
C. Intraaortic balloon pump	___ Treatment of aberrant impulses
D. Intracoronary stent	___ Muscle flap used to reinforce damaged heart muscle
E. Extracorporeal oxygenation	___ Removal of plaque from the arterial wall
F. Cryoablation	___ Revascularize the myocardium
G. Ventricular aneurysmectomy	___ Treatment for end-stage myocardial disease
H. Cardiomyoplasty	___ Percutaneous transluminal coronary angioplasty
I. Angioplasty	___ Provides structural support for coronary arteries
J. Cardiac transplant	___ Assist ventricular function

CRITICAL THINKING ACTIVITIES

Create a case study about a patient in end-stage cardiac failure. Describe the surgical options and the assistive devices used to sustain life until definitive treatment is performed. Identify the expected outcomes and evaluate the simulated plan of care.

CHAPTER 40 — PERIPHERAL VASCULAR SURGERY

LEARNING OBJECTIVES

- Identify the pertinent anatomy of ateriovascular system.
- Understand the potential complications associated with peripheral vascular disease.
- Describe the handling and preparation of vascular grafts used for peripheral vascular surgery.

STUDY QUESTIONS

1. List several risk factors for developing peripheral vascular disease.
2. Atherosclerosis is a principle factor of what disease processes?
3. What is the action of fibrinolytic therapy?
4. What are the most serious complications of peripheral vascular surgery that require immediate return to the OR?
5. What is the advantage of using autologous saphenous vein graft?
6. Describe the preparation of a synthetic graft prosthesis for use in a patient.
7. What is a potential serious complication of carotid endarterectomy?
8. What is the major concern of clamping the aorta when repairing an aortic aneurysm?
9. Describe the phenomena of pulmonary emboli.
10. What measures can be taken when anticoagulant therapy has failed or is not indicated for thromboembolic disease of the lower extremities or pelvis?

MATCHING: Each letter is used only once.

Procedure	Definition
A. Embolectomy	___ Obstruction is vaporized
B. Atherectomy	___ Prosthetic to maintain patency after dilation of vessel
C. Balloon dilation	___ Removal of traveling blood clot
D. Intraluminal stent	___ Plaque is pulverized by a high speed burr
E. Laser angioplasty	___ Compresses atheromatous material against arterial wall
F. Fibrinolytic therapy	___ Removal of stationary blood clot
G. Thrombectomy	___ Pharmacologic injection to maintain patency after dilation of vessel

CRITICAL THINKING ACTIVITIES

Create a case study about a patient who has had progressive carotid stenosis for several years. Include consideration for age and general health status of the patient. Identify the expected outcomes and evaluate the simulated plan of care.

SECTION ELEVEN: *MULTIDISCIPLINARY PERIOPERATIVE CONSIDERATIONS*

Multidisciplinary considerations include specific patient populations, such as patients who qualify for ambulatory status, pediatric patients, geriatric patients, organ donors and transplant recipients, and cancer patients. These specific patient populations have been identified to have common intrinsic characteristics within identifiable groups that should be routinely considered during the development of the plan of care. These patient populations can be compared, in part, to the *Patient with Special Needs* in Chapter 8. The main contrast of multidisciplinary considerations and special needs patients is demonstrated in life-stage issues, medical diagnoses, surgical complexity, and potential for negative outcomes. Patients with special needs associated with medical diagnoses, such as pregnancy, diabetes, or morbid obesity can be found within many age groups and patient populations.

CHAPTER 41 — AMBULATORY SURGERY

LEARNING OBJECTIVES

- Compare the differences between hospital-based surgical services and free-standing surgical services.
- Compare the flow of patient care between one day stay and full admission status.
- Identify patient eligibility criteria for ambulatory surgery status.
- Compare the advantages and disadvantages of ambulatory surgery.
- Understand the importance of postoperative teaching for the success of the ambulatory process.

STUDY QUESTIONS

1. Describe the main differences between ambulatory surgery admission and full in-house admission status.
2. List the most common reasons for an ambulatory patient's postoperative admission to a free-standing recovery care center or hospital.
3. List the criteria for eligibility for ambulatory surgery.
4. Outline an overview of pre- and postoperative instructions for a patient having an ambulatory surgical procedure.
5. What are the benefits of a postoperative phone call to the patient after discharge?
6. Documentation of ambulatory surgical care should include:
7. Give five examples of settings where patients are admitted, have a surgical procedure, and are discharged on the same day.
8. List several examples of surgical procedures that are safely performed in ambulatory surgery settings.

9. Compare several advantages and disadvantages of ambulatory surgery.
10. List several criteria for patient discharge from an ambulatory surgery facility.

CRITICAL THINKING ACTIVITIES

Diagram two separate patient care scenarios. The first scenario should describe total ambulatory care including the personnel, facility type, and services involved from admission to discharge. The second scenario should describe, in contrast, total in-house patient care of a nonambulatory patient including 24-hour patient care personnel, facility layout, and services involved from admission to discharge.

CHAPTER 42 — PERIOPERATIVE PEDIATRICS

LEARNING OBJECTIVES

- Describe specific considerations for pediatric patient care according to each developmental stage.
- Identify physiologic differences by age that influence the development of the plan of care.
- Identify psychologic differences by age that influence the plan of care.
- List several procedures performed exclusively on pediatric patients.

STUDY QUESTIONS

1. Neonates born before completion of 37 weeks gestation are referred to as:
2. Fetal viability is based on what criteria?
3. Psychologic considerations of the pediatric patient's plan of care are based on:
4. List several congenital anomalies that would be incompatible with life if not corrected by surgery.
5. What is the leading cause of death in children?
6. What are several key elements of fluid and electrolyte balance in a pediatric patient?
7. List several methods of body temperature monitoring and regulation in a pediatric patient.
8. What are three causes of heat loss for any patient?
9. What are several indicators of pain perception in a pediatric patient?
10. List several safety considerations for the perioperative care of a pediatric patient.

CRITICAL THINKING ACTIVITIES

Create a pediatric plan of care for one specific age group undergoing a specific surgical procedure. Select a developmental stage theorist who has developed and researched theories specifically related to the age group selected. Combine psychologic and physiologic factors found in the developmental theory in simulating assessment, nursing diagnoses, and intervention factors. The plan should include consideration of the parent's or guardian's needs also. Identify key expected outcomes and evaluate the plan of care.

CHAPTER 43   PERIOPERATIVE GERIATRICS

LEARNING OBJECTIVES

- Understand how comorbidity influences the care of the gerontologic patient.
- Identify several theories of aging.
- Discuss how cultural considerations impact psychologic aspects of aging.
- Discuss several myths about aging.
- Identify specific features of perioperative geriatric patient care.

STUDY QUESTIONS

1. Define comorbidity.
2. How does comorbidity impact the perioperative geriatric patient?
3. Preoperative assessment may take longer with a geriatric patient because:
4. List several intraoperative considerations for the geriatric patient.
5. Name three influences on the way in which an individual ages.
6. Describe how culture influences the psychosocial aspects of aging.
7. Wound healing may be complicated in the elderly patient because:
8. Explain the significance of preoperative assessment of functional ability in the elderly.
9. What is the impact of psychosocial isolation in the elderly?
10. Postoperative assessment of the elderly patient should include:

CRITICAL THINKING ACTIVITIES

Create a geriatric plan of care for a specific surgical procedure. Consideration for pre- and postoperative assessment, preparation, and positioning should be included. Combine psychologic and physiologic factors found in the developmental theory in simulating assessment, nursing diagnoses, and intervention factors. Identify key expected outcomes and evaluate the plan of care.

CHAPTER 44   ORGAN PROCUREMENT, TRANSPLANTATION, REPLANTATION

LEARNING OBJECTIVES

- Identify specific criteria which should be met for organ donation.
- List brain death criteria for organ donation.
- Understand the roles of procurement and transplant team members.
- Understand the roles of the host facility scrub person and circulator in organ procurement and transplantation.
- Describe the psychologic impact of organ donation on the family of the donor.
- Describe the psychologic impact of organ procurement on operating room caregivers.

STUDY QUESTIONS

1. What are three important goals of transplantation?
2. A patient with HIV or HBV may receive an allograft. TRUE / FALSE
3. What are some of the indications for a bone marrow transplant?
4. List several types of tissue that can be transplanted from one person to another and function normally.
5. What Act is recognized by all 50 states as a legal consent for organ donation?
6. If a deceased person has not signed a donor card, their family may not be approached for possible tissue and organ donation. TRUE / FALSE.
7. What biologic functions are maintained in a heartbeating cadaver donor before and during organ procurement?
8. What organs can be procured from nonheartbeating donors?
9. Who pays for tissue and organ procurement?
10. Procured organs are placed in sterile containers and packed with dry ice to decrease ischemia. TRUE / FALSE
11. Tissue-typing is the detection of what substance known to affect rejection?
12. Which two components of the immune system appear to be responsible for rejection?
13. How is a donor evaluated for a heart transplant?
14. Which immunosuppressive drug, given preoperatively, enhances healing and combats cell-mediated rejection in heart-lung and lung transplants?
15. A living, related donor may give a kidney or a lobe of liver or lung to another person who is a tissue match. TRUE / FALSE
16. What are some major goals for having a pancreas transplant?
17. Transportation of a traumatically amputated part includes preservation of the part by what means?
18. Assessment of a patient who has suffered traumatic amputation should include:
19. List several physical structures that are repaired and/or anastomosed during replantation of an amputated part.
20. What are some of the contraindications for replantation of an amputated part?

MATCHING: Each letter is used only once.

Transplanted Tissue		Definition
A. Allografts	___	Genetically identical donor and recipient
B. Autografts	___	Transplants to an anatomically abnormal location
C. Isografts	___	Homograft, genetically different humans
D. Xenografts	___	Transplant to normal recipient site
E. Orthotopic transplants	___	Donor is recipient
F. Heterotopic transplants	___	Tissue grafted between different species

MATCHING: Each letter is used only once.

Type of rejection		Time frame of rejection and prognosis
A. Hyperacute	___	Within 5 days, transplanted organ is removed
B. Accelerated	___	Insidious onset, not reversible
C. Acute	___	Within 24 hours, transplanted organ is removed
D. Chronic	___	Between 1 week to 4 months, sometimes reversible

CRITICAL THINKING ACTIVITIES

Create a case study about a family involved with a living-related donor and recipient. Include age-related developmental data for both the donor and recipient. Pre-, intra-, and postoperative assessment considerations should be included in the plan of care. Identify and evaluate the attainment of expected outcomes.

CHAPTER 45   ONCOLOGY

LEARNING OBJECTIVES

- Identify the clinical signs and symptoms of cancer.
- Understand the standard criteria for classification of tumors.
- Understand the factors that may predispose the patient to cancer.
- Describe the role of radiation therapy in the treatment and/or palliation of cancer.
- List several common areas of carcinoma in situ.
- List several forms of adjunctive therapy in the treatment of cancer.
- List several procedures used to diagnose cancer in the operating room.
- Identify the hazards associated with the treatment of cancer.
- Understand the psychosocial impact of the diagnosis of cancer.

STUDY QUESTIONS

1. What is the atypical new growth of abnormal cells or tissues, which may be malignant or benign?
2. List the clinical warning signs and symptoms of cancer.
3. What do the initials TNMR mean in tumor classification?
4. Lymphadenectomy is performed as a prophylaxis to inhibit the spread of cancer. TRUE / FALSE
5. List 3 types of infusion catheters used for cancer chemotherapy.
6. Explain why tissue specimens are not placed in formalin when further evaluation is needed to determine course of treatment.
7. List several areas of the body where interstitial radiation sources are implanted.
8. What safety precautions are followed when handling radiation sources?
9. List several toxic side effects of chemotherapy:
10. What steps are taken to combat malnutrition?

MATCH THE TREATMENT WITH THE METHOD IN WHICH THE TREATMENT WORKS. Each letter is used only once.

TREATMENT	PHYSIOLOGY OF TREATMENT
A. Endocrine therapy	____ Tissue-oxygen molecules destroy tumor cells
B. Photodynamic therapy	____ Cellular metabolism is affected by specific hormone receptors
C. Radiation therapy	____ Interruption of cell life cycle
D. Chemotherapy	____ Positive and negative ions affect metabolic activity of cells

CRITICAL THINKING ACTIVITIES

Create a case study about a patient with cancer of a major organ. Diagram potential routes of metastasis and the impact on other organ systems. Describe the perioperative plan of care including diagnostics, interventions, and postoperative follow-up. Consideration should be given to psychosocial and developmental issues surrounding the diagnosis of cancer. The family and/or significant others should be included in the plan. Identify and evaluate the attainment of expected outcomes.